"This is a comprehensive approach to ...
. . . Lose It For Life isn't just about ...
the abundant life the Good Shepherd promises to all His sheep."

"I've decided I will not pay the price for the sins of others and that I truly desire the best for me. Thanks for getting me on the path and telling me the truth that I will have to persevere. Mostly thank you for your love and the hope you've given me to create a new life for myself."

"Thank you for helping me find the grace and peace which God has given freely and I never accepted until now. I did not realize until last night that I had not surrendered the pain and anger of my daughter's death. Now I have, and I am free of that hiding in my body."

"LIFL changed my life and my thinking about diets and my weight. I know I am not alone and can now face the future and make some needed changes."

"I CAN keep it off, and I CAN make positive and gradual changes in my life! The biggest change for me has been to my goal—from just losing weight to living a truly healthy life."

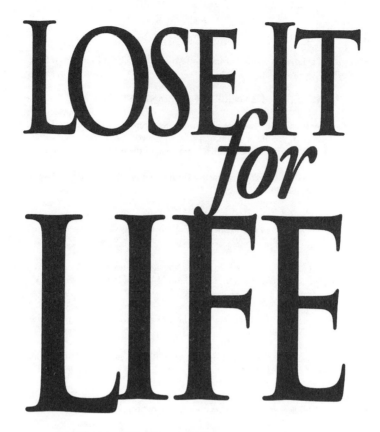

LOSE IT *for* LIFE

THE TOTAL SOLUTION
—SPIRITUAL, EMOTIONAL, PHYSICAL—
FOR PERMANENT WEIGHT LOSS

STEPHEN ARTERBURN, M.ED.
DR. LINDA MINTLE

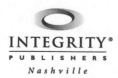

INTEGRITY®
PUBLISHERS
Nashville

Lose It for Life

Copyright © 2004 by Stephen Arterburn and Linda Mintle.

Published by Integrity Publishers, a division of Integrity Media, Inc., 5250 Virginia Way, Suite 110, Brentwood, TN 37027.

HELPING PEOPLE WORLDWIDE EXPERIENCE the MANIFEST PRESENCE of GOD.

All rights reserved. No portion of this book may be reproduced, stored in a retrieval system, or transmitted in any form or by any means—electronic, mechanical, photocopy, recording, or any other—except for brief quotations in printed reviews, without the prior written permission of the publisher.

Stephen Arterburn published in association with Alive Communications, 7680 Goddard Street, Suite 200, Colorado Springs, Colorado 80920.

Unless otherwise noted, Scripture quotations are taken from the Holy Bible, New International Version®, NIV®. Copyright © 1973, 1978, 1984 by the International Bible Society. Used by permission of Zondervan. All rights reserved.

Scripture quotations designated MSG are taken from The Message by Eugene H. Peterson. Copyright © 1993, 1994, 1995, 1996, 2000, 2001, 2002. Used by permission of NavPress Publishing Group. All rights reserved.

Scripture quotations marked NASB are from the New American Standard Bible. Copyright © 1960, 1962, 1963, 1968, 1971, 1972, 1973, 1975, 1977 by the Lockman Foundation. Used by permission. All rights reserved.

Scripture quotations designated NLT are taken from The Holy Bible: New Living Translation. Copyright © 1986 by Tyndale House Publishers. Wheaton, Illinois, 60189. Used by permission. All rights reserved.

Scripture quotations designated TLB are taken from The Living Bible by Kenneth N. Taylor. Copyright © 1971. Tyndale House Publishers, Inc. Used by permission. All rights reserved.

Scripture quotations designated NKJV are taken from the Holy Bible, New King James Version. Thomas Nelson Publishers, Nashville, TN. Copyright © 1982. Used by permission. All rights reserved.

Scripture quotations designated AMP are taken from The Amplified Bible, Old Testament, copyright © 1965, 1987 by the Zondervan Corporation and The Amplified Bible, New Testament, copyright © 1958, 1987 by The Lockman Foundation. Used by permission. All rights reserved.

Scripture quotations designated KJV are taken from the Holy Bible, King James Version.

This book is not intended to provide therapy, counseling, clinical advice or treatment or to take the place of clinical advice and treatment from your personal physician or professional mental health provider. Readers are advised to consult their own qualified healthcare physician regarding mental health or medical issues. Neither the publisher nor the author takes any responsibility for any possible consequences from any treatment, action or application of information in this book to the reader.

Cover Design: Brand Navigation, LLC (Bill Chiaravalle, Mark Mickel); brandnavigation.com
Cover Image: Steve Gardner, PixelWorks
Interior: Sharon Collins/Artichoke Design

ISBN 1-59145-245-7

Printed in the United States of America
07 08 RRD 9 8 7 6 5 4 3

This is dedicated to the over 1,000 Losers who have attended the Lose It For Life Institute. Thank you for helping me shape this material into what it is today. And thanks for staying in touch and connected.

CONTENTS

GETTING STARTED

If you are struggling to lose weight or keep off pounds already lost, you are in good company. Obesity is a veritable epidemic in our society. Nearly 65 percent of American adults (or more than 120 million people) are considered overweight or obese.[1] And despite billions of dollars spent on countless diet books and health products, we Americans are more overweight than ever.

To be *overweight* or *obese* means to have a medical condition caused by an excess of body fat. By general definition, you are overweight if your body mass index (BMI) is between 25-29.9; obese if it is above 30.[2] And while these terms can be easily defined and measured through a number of techniques, most of us need only look in the mirror or stand on the scale to know if we are in trouble.

Samuel Klein, president of the North American Association for the Study of Obesity, notes that technically advanced societies with an abundance of food and sedentary lifestyles are especially at risk for producing overweight people.[3] The speed at which this is happening in America is reason for concern. If you are like most people, you are probably trying to lose weight right now, or you are at least thinking about it. And while losing weight seems like an uphill battle in which the mountain is never fully climbed, it is in truth a battle that can be won.

It is our hope that this book is the last one you'll ever have to read concerning the topic of weight loss. We know most of you have stacks of books you've purchased over the years that detail all sorts of angles and fads for shedding unwanted pounds. Each of those diet books represents your good intentions to conquer that mountain. But for reasons only you know, you haven't won the battle . . . yet.

Perhaps you know someone who is losing weight on the fad diet of the day, or maybe you are trying yourself. After a while, were you right back where you started or in even worse shape than before? It's a familiar story, and it's likely that you are reading this book with a bit of mistrust or skepticism. Let us reassure you that it's okay. We aren't here to help you embark upon another failure. We don't want to promise hope and not deliver. We want you to be successful—to lose weight for life.

Actually, losing weight isn't really the issue. Your closet full of multiple-sized clothing is testimony to the number of times you've lost and gained weight in your lifetime. Some of you are experts at weight loss and could write your own books about your experiences: eating grapefruits, downing vats of "fat burning" cabbage soup, consuming liquid shakes, protein bars, low-fat brownies, and low-carb ice cream. Our personal favorite is the diet in which you lose weight by breathing differently. It's enough to make us all crazy!

We Americans are tempted by quick fixes. The problem with quick weight-loss ideas is that they don't work for very long and require drastic changes in the way we eat—changes which are impossible to maintain over time. Some fad diets are even dangerous and can lead to serious health problems. Recently, I (Steve) was sitting in an airport with Byron Williamson, president, and Joey Paul, senior vice president, of my publisher. We were reviewing the cover for this book when the woman at the table next to us overheard our conversation. She wanted to know which diet we thought was the best and asked if Lose It For Life was a healthy plan. She explained that she had just quit a diet because of her health. Though she had lost weight, her cholesterol was at 148 and manageable when she started the diet. However, after only a short time she was forced to take medication to get her cholesterol under control and had to stop using that particular diet. She is only one of many who have hurt their health while trying to lose weight the wrong way.

The real issue isn't *if* you can lose weight. You can. But can you lose weight sensibly and keep it off? Can you lose it for life? The answer to both questions is yes.

There is no foolproof diet. Look around. For all our obsession with weight-loss gimmicks, we continue to experience record rates of obesity. We must change our lifestyles, learn to eat sensibly, and exercise. This doesn't sound exciting or terribly new, but it is a long-term strategy that works. And this book can help you make change happen. We encourage you to try again if you have struggled or failed with other methods of weight loss. And if this is your first time trying to lose weight, welcome! We'll share what we know from both personal and clinical experience.

I, Steve, used to weigh sixty pounds more than I do today. I know the heartache of losing the weight, feeling great, and then losing control and gaining it all back. I know how it feels to essentially carry around the equivalent of a third grader on my person. And I know the horror of another approaching summer when everyone will be in a swimsuit and I will have no place to hide.

For years I felt like a second-class citizen because I was fatter than any of my friends. But I was more than that. I was unhealthy. My blood pressure was so high that I was on medication while I was still in my early twenties. I was out of breath and out of energy most of the time. I couldn't run around the block, even at a slow jog! I was facing an early death. And just like you, I had a brain that functioned . . . my weight problem was not a result of lacking IQ points. The problem went deeper; it was emotional and it was spiritual. There was within me a stubborn resistance to do what would eventually change my life.

For a long time, I counted on my troubled mind that got me into trouble to get me out of trouble. I tried the same old tactics over and over again, only to fail over and over again. But fortunately, I awoke one day sick and tired of being sick and tired. My life was never to be the same again. I had experienced a spiritual awakening that led to a new willingness to change. Based on those changes, I developed the Lose It For Life plan—not a diet, but a plan that can work with any diet. Not a behavioral plan that leads to a temporary change in the way you look, but a healthy plan to address spiritual and emotional needs at the core of your being.

The Lose It For Life plan is really a strategy for a healthy life. I have been living by it for years, and the results on my own life have been profound. I have seen what poor eating habits can do to a person. My father was a great man, but he didn't know how to eat. His cholesterol was horrible, and he was on blood-pressure medication, just as I was in my early twenties. He died at sixty-eight of a massive heart attack. It broke my heart because I had so many plans for us over the years that would have followed. Though I was a sitting duck for the same health problems, I gave up some old family eating patterns and adopted the Lose It For Life plan.

So far so good. I just had an annual checkup and my blood work was fantastic. Not one indicator was above or below normal. And the indicators for heart disease showed that I was at one-fourth the risk for heart disease compared to other males my age. I look forward to a long future, and I hope to one day hear that you have experienced the same results.

These radical life changes began from a spiritual place within me— a place of surrender that led me to a new willingness to do whatever it took to get the weight off. I began to lose the weight and have kept it off for over twenty years. That same willingness to learn and heal and change is the same willingness I try to instill in the hearts of those people who attend the Lose It For Life Institute I have conducted bi-annually for the past few years. People have paid $1,600 to attend the conference and often had to buy two airline seats to come (that was just for one person!). Many have tried everything; some are on their third gastric bypass surgery. But even after having paid all of that money and going to all the trouble to attend, they often come with little willingness to change.

By the end of the five-day experience, there is real change and they are on a different path. We have followed up with attendants to discover that many do lose weight. I have learned much from those who attend these institutes. Others haven't lost weight but have changed their lives and are actually living for the first time. And sadly, there are also those who make no changes and continue down the same path as before.

Lose It For Life is the culmination of a lifelong journey of first having a weight problem, then finding a way to be free of it for life, and sharing the method of that victory with others. I also bring with me thirty years of experience of working with fellow strugglers of all types of addiction and dependency.

And I, Dr. Linda, bring over twenty years of personal experience working with clients' eating disorders and food and weight problems. Over the years, I've worked with hundreds of people who have tried all kinds of diets, felt the agony of defeat, been stigmatized because of their weight, endured shame and humiliation due to their size, and felt hope-less in terms of overcoming the compulsion to overeat.

I've consulted with low-calorie diet programs, completed pre-surgical evaluations for patients considering surgical treatment for obesity, and been instrumental in reviewing medication options for patients. I have spent countless hours with patients in individual, marital, family, and group therapy sessions for eating disorders, including those struggling with compulsive overeating and binge eating. All that to say, I've heard your stories and witnessed the tremendous effort you have put forth to lose weight.

Personally, I struggled with my own weight during a traumatic time in my life. Following the death of my oldest brother, I unconsciously used food to soothe my cycling emotional state and deal with his passing. At the time, I had no idea that my eating was connected to my emotional pain. My training as a therapist and faith in God helped me make this connection and gradually lose the excess thirty pounds. I have maintained that weight loss for twenty years.

We intend to be practical, helpful, insightful, and spiritually alert. We want you to be successful, and we want to help you lose weight without feeling shame, guilt, pressure, or condemnation. Though the weight-loss journey isn't easy, it is possible to lose weight and keep it off. You *can* lose weight for life.

Lose It For Life (LIFL) is not about dieting. It's not about exercising, although exercise does play a part. There is no quick fix, magical diet, or even the promise of a thin body. Losing weight and keeping it off has more to do with changing how you think, feel, and act at any given moment rather than what you eat or whether you take part in a regular exercise program. Lose It For Life is about creating a *lifestyle* of permanent weight management that emphasizes the whole you: your spirit, mind, body, and emotions. It is about discovering meaningful connections with others, support, and community.

Spiritual renewal and transformation, an important part of LIFL, are not typically part of weight-loss programs. Yet without both, you will struggle to keep weight off. It is through a deeper relationship with God and others that hope and encouragement will flood your soul.

When you read the word "spiritual," what do you picture? Do you envision an angry fundamentalist who throws rules and regulations at you while grinning with insincerity? Or perhaps you think we speak of some esoteric experience that no one ever really "gets." If you can relate to either of these scenarios, you're in for a pleasant surprise. We want to help you understand authentic spirituality, and also to examine why the counterfeit of that very thing may be keeping you fat. You are a physical being, and a diet might help you address that. But you are also a spiritual person from the inside out, and it is in that core of you that the battle is fought and then either won or lost. We are going to help you with that spiritual battle.

Have you ever found yourself saying, "All I have to do to lose weight is . . . "? It's a common lie that most all of us who have struggled with weight have told ourselves—that if we change just one thing, the weight will go away. We want to believe that there is a simple solution to our very complex problem, but there isn't. Instead, there are many variables within your own personal equation to consider. With the help of this book, and by combining the necessary components to maintain your weight-management lifestyle, you will form a personal plan for living a healthier life.

Be encouraged, because you can lose it for life! There are so many positive reasons to go forward! Losing it for life is exciting and completely possible. Commit to these ten positive reasons to begin this journey as you:

1. Improve your health. As you gain a proper view of food and nutrition and become more active, you will lose excess pounds. Research shows that even losing a small amount of weight can bring physical benefit!

2. Accept God's free gift of grace and become less judgmental

as you are freed of your own guilt and shame.

3. Become defined by who you are, not what you weigh.

4. Gain an awareness of the difference between physical, emotional, and spiritual hunger—and learn ways to satisfy all three.

5. Find yourself more in tune with your body as you accept God's design for you as good.

6. Take your negative thoughts captive, renew your mind, and think in more positive ways.

7. Assume responsibility for your behavior and lose the victim position.

8. Practice managing your emotions instead of allowing them to manage you. Emotions won't be frightening as you learn to confront them head-on and work through the pain.

9. Make new and healthy connections with others—an important part of your recovery.

10. Learn how to preserve spiritual gains and persevere to the finish.

PART ONE

SEVEN KEYS TO LOSE IT FOR LIFE

SURRENDER

ACCEPTANCE

CONFESSION

RESPONSIBILITY

FORGIVENESS

TRANSFORMATION

PRESERVATION

At one time we too were foolish, disobedient, deceived and enslaved by all kinds of passions and pleasures. . . . But when the kindness and love of God our Savior appeared, he saved us, not because of righteous things we had done, but because of his mercy.

— TITUS 3:3-5

1
What Do You Have to Lose?

Food is everywhere! Enticing ads fill the pages of magazines. Billboards loaded with images of pizzas and burgers grab our attention. Television commercials lure us to the refrigerator in search of late-night, feel-good snacks. And if we really want to be scintillated, we can tune in to an entire television network dedicated to scrumptious food preparation, as well as experiencing (however vicariously) the ecstasy associated with eating those specialties. Anyone who is triggered to eat by the mere mention of food or easy access to it is in big trouble in this snack-infested, food-congested society of ours.

Hurried schedules give way to too many fast food meals eaten on the go. And fast food almost always means fat food. Portions are super-sized and a bargain to boot. Some authorities insist that much of our society's obesity comes from one source: Carbonated soft drinks—a fancy name for flavored sugar water—are consumed in vat-like 32- to 64-ounce containers called "Big Gulps®" and "Giant Swallows®." High prices discourage the purchase of organic and whole foods, fresh fruits, and vegetables. Public high schools subsidize their funding by placing soda and snack machines in their halls of learning. And school lunches are filled with nutritionally bankrupt food.

The food industry isn't solely to blame for amplifying our problem with food. The multi-billion dollar fashion industry promotes an ideal body image that is nearly impossible to replicate, so we give up and collapse into the extreme opposite of the ideal. Guilt and shame glare back from the mirror as we camouflage our thighs and secretly purchase cellulite-reducing creams. Thanks to media, any chance for a healthy body image is gone before puberty hits. Food becomes our enemy and our lover, truly a relationship as complicated as any other.

When it comes to eating, American culture is toxic. As consumers, we are encouraged to ignore the consequences of overindulgence and our mentality of always needing more. Among the "You deserve a break today™" mantras, the messages are consistent: You are entitled to what you want, and you should be immediately gratified (whenever you wish!). However, giving in to these hedonistic messages has led to a serious fall out. As a country, we are fatter than ever and playing roulette with our physical health, mental health, and spiritual lives. Our sedentary lifestyles, combined with a poor diet, have led to an obesity epidemic.

American culture promises satisfaction from the pursuit of pleasure. Yet one of the richest and wisest kings of all time (Solomon) concluded that chasing pleasure as an end unto itself only leads to despair. When we lose sight of the Giver of all pleasure (food, taste, and eating included), we carry a burden of excess, both physically and spiritually.

Even the church culture can add to our difficulties. So much of what goes on outside of a Sunday service, most of the social opportunities of the church, in fact, revolve around food. Surely the potluck was invented in a church somewhere in the Midwest. It is almost as if we look for occasions to get together and eat. Additionally, we hear sermons about the evils of alcohol, drugs, and sex outside of marriage, but we seldom hear the Word on gluttony. In fact, some of the best Christian speakers have never resolved their own food issues, so they do not address them with their followers. They would be fired if they entered the pulpit drunk, drugged, or holding a pornographic magazine, but they are excused from taking an extra two hundred pounds up onto the platform. They scream an unspoken message that food is the one acceptable addiction of the church.

In society at large, there is a strange dichotomy surrounding food and weight. Our culture simultaneously encourages gorging at the fast food trough and the all-you-can-stuff buffets, while also frowning deeply on those who pack on extra pounds and look anything less than walking advertisements for anorexia. It is an unwritten American eleventh commandment: Thou shalt not be fat. Yet, like the original Law, we are living evidence that this commandment cannot be carried out in our own power. With more than 120 million overweight people,[4] another 5–10 million suffering from eating disorders, and still another 25 million suffering from binge-eating disorders,[5] more than willpower is involved in this battle.

The cultural vilification of overweight people guarantees we will try anything to escape the stigma. The billion-dollar dieting industry plays us like a fine violin. When we aren't feeling momentarily defeated, we will embrace another gimmick and believe in its power even when the claims defy all logic. Our sensibilities are lost on the fact that if any of these dieting schemes actually worked, all serious weight-loss programs would go out of business.

But desperation leads to drastic measures—we will try anything for the promise of becoming the incredible shrinking woman or man. The industry knows this and persuades us to keep trying to be thin. And if we buy into the seduction, we can live our lives chasing false images perpetuated by the media. Witness the horror and fascination on MTV as people spend thousands of dollars and suffer intense pain under the knives of plastic surgeons in order to have their frames and faces remade to physically look like famous stars they idolize. What isn't often shown to the general public are the horror stories of such procedures. A recent television story shared the despair of a mother whose daughter choked to death on her own blood while she recovered from a liposuction procedure in the office of a local plastic surgeon. Truly, does a sixteen-year-old really need to undergo such a surgery in order to live a happy and fulfilled life?

And we forget, or never realize, that our spiritual connection to a loving heavenly Father offers real help and truth without distortion in a way no advertiser or program could ever deliver. Dissatisfied and unhappy with life, the hope is that external beauty will translate into opportunity, acceptance, and new life. But as the book of Ecclesiastes reminds us, this is vanity and only leads to emptiness. Lasting happiness and a rich and fulfilling life will only be found in a right relationship with God and others.

So what's the message? *This culture is not going to endorse your decision to change.* It will not help you control your eating nor offer friendly support. In fact, it may oppose the very measures that contribute to you successfully losing weight for life. But there is reason to hope. In the midst of all the negative influences of our food-saturated society and weight-conscious culture, there is another message: It is possible to lose weight and keep it off.

Seven Keys[6] to Lose It For Life

1. SURRENDER. "So humble yourselves under the mighty power of God, and in his good time he will honor you" (1 Peter 5:6 NLT). You must be willing to discover what is driving the hunger and want healing more than you want food. You are unable to accomplish your goals without relinquishing control and surrendering to His way of doing things.

2. ACCEPTANCE. "O LORD, you have examined my heart and know everything about me" (Psalm 139:1 NLT). You must be determined to face and own the emo-

---

tional issues, pain, and loss that you uncover behind the hunger. Accept the reality of your weight and the need for help. Stay in the reality of your life, accepting your need for help. God sees your heart. He knows your need and will provide the help you require.

3. CONFESSION. "Confess your sins to each other and pray for each other so that you may be healed" (James 5:16 NLT). Come out of hiding. Open up to God and others about the reality of your struggles. While it is often difficult to admit your shortcomings and areas of weakness, it is what keeps us honest and real with each other. Confession truly is good for the soul. You must find people you can trust who can handle your secrets and help you heal.

4. RESPONSIBILITY. "For we are each responsible for our own conduct" (Galatians 6:5 NLT). Taking responsibility for change, moving out of the victim position, and owning up to your mistakes is necessary to lose it for life. When you are hurt or experience loss, it's easy to blame others or feel like a victim. However, you must believe that God will bring purpose and meaning out of pain, and then you must move on.

5. FORGIVENESS. "If you forgive those who sin against you, your heavenly Father will forgive you" (Matthew 6:14 NLT). Forgive your own failures and the failures of those who have hurt you. Forgiveness is not optional in the Christian life and yet many of us hold on to bitterness and wonder why we don't experience joy and other benefits of the Christian life. When you give up grudges and make restitution for past wrongs, you experience spiritual blessings.

6. TRANSFORMATION. "All praise to the God and Father of our Lord Jesus Christ. He is the source of every mercy and the God who comforts us. He comforts us in all our troubles so that we can comfort others. When others are troubled, we will be able to give them the same comfort God has given us" (2 Corinthians 1:3-4 NLT). Transform your struggle, pain, and loss into a purposeful mission. God's way is to take those things you have suffered and use them for His glory. Out of pain and difficulty come compassion for others and a willingness to reach out because of the grace and mercy shown to you.

7. PRESERVATION. "So make every effort to apply the benefits of these promises to your life. Then your faith will produce a life of moral excellence. A life of moral excellence leads to knowing God better" (2 Peter 1:5 NLT). Perseverance is required to make it through life's inevitable struggles and keep the spiritual gains made. When you discover the signs and phases of relapse, you will learn to maintain your weight loss for life.

Control or Surrender?

Life is difficult. Just when we think we have things under control, something happens to remind us that control is elusive. The children who brought such pleasure early on now bring headaches and heartbreaks with rebellion and even rejection. The promotion at work gives you more money but robs you of valuable time and peace of mind. The truth is, we aren't really in control. And until we come to terms with this reality, our lives are destined to be full of anxiety, fear of the future, guilt over the past, and anger at others. Notice—each of these is an excuse to eat!

We can, however, pretend to be in control, especially when it comes to losing weight. We pretend by lying to ourselves about the quick fix that fixes nothing or the instant solution that only makes matters worse. We delude ourselves with the mantras of all those who have failed before us:

· All I have to do is have more willpower.

· All I have to do is just stop eating so much.

· All I have to do is quit being so lazy and exercise more.

· All I have to do is take more control of my life.

· I can do anything if I try hard enough.

And when I no longer believe the lie that I can do whatever I set my mind to, I succumb to the opposite extreme, believing I can do nothing and all is hopeless. The murmurs of my aching soul are:

· My weight is genetic and there is nothing I can do about it.

· It's a sin to dig up the past—what's done is done.

· If I was supposed to be thin, I would have been born that way.

We beat our heads against that same brick wall many times before we realize that our own power is not getting us very far. Check your head. I bet there are many bruises! If so, it's time for a change.

Rather than fight with the same ineffective weapons that have backfired so many times, why not surrender this battle for weight loss? Pull out the white flag and vigorously wave it. Give yourself over to a higher authority; relinquish control to God. He can be trusted, especially when we feel weak and defeated. As the apostle Paul reminds us, "When I am weak, then I am strong (2 Corinthians 12:10). In fact, when we come to the end of ourselves, God is waiting to step in and provide rest for the weary, and chances are you could use a little reprieve from this exhausting fight. After all, what do you have to lose?

Why not give up the illusion of control and yield to God's mercy and grace? In 1 Peter 5:6 Paul tells us, "So humble yourselves under the mighty power of God, and in his good time he will honor you" (NLT). Acknowledge your weakness and invite God into the process. Accept the radical notion that if you could have fixed your weight problem on your own, under your own power, you would have done it by now and the struggle would be over. You have to make an admission. You have to admit you cannot handle this on your own. You have to admit that God can. And you have to let Him do this work, even if it means working with God's people to accomplish the transformation that is necessary (it will!). When you let go of your life and put it into God's hands, you are in good hands.

God is the Creator of all life and the Lord of the universe. But since the Garden of Eden, men and women have continually played God and tried unsuccessfully to rule over their own destinies. From Genesis through Revelation, Scripture reveals humankind's natural incapacity to live healthy, God-pleasing lives. The Old Testament describes a colorful assortment of characters who turned their backs on God's ways and inevitably experienced fear, foolishness, and failure. Fortunately, some of them surrendered to the ultimate power of God, allowing Him to intervene in their lives with divine power and wisdom. In the New Testament, Christ's death on the cross made God's intervention even more accessible—He took upon Himself the willfulness and rebellion of the entire world. His resurrection brought hope for new life.

Through years of failed weight loss attempts, the road of self-effort and control has not taken you where you wanted to go. Proverbs 14:12 tells us, "Before every man there lies a wide and pleasant road that seems right but ends in death" (TLB). To stay on this road is to choose further heartache and destruction. Consequently, we must be willing to admit that our lives have spun out of control. Self-control and our forms of self-treatment have failed us and must be abandoned.

Although we are limited by our weaknesses, God is not. By acknowledging that He alone has the power to change the course of our lives, we surrender to Him our powerlessness and begin the process of spiritual renewal. Only when we relinquish our control to God does He release His supernatural power in our lives, and it is only through His power that we can be transformed by the renewing of our minds (Romans 12:2).

Every limitation we have can be seen as an invitation from God to do for us what we cannot do for ourselves. When we surrender, we don't just give up or play dead or wait for God to fix us. Instead, we become active participants with God in making a new path of hope toward healing. We drop our guard and give up our solitary and isolated efforts to heal. We sincerely and humbly reach out to others who can help us restore our lives to spiritual vitality. Surrender is not passivity, nor is it resignation. Its motion requires an active and conscious turning toward God wherein we reflect our willingness to submit to His power by living out our newfound truth and sharing it with others.

Surrender means:

· humbling ourselves before the God of the universe.

· admitting that God is all powerful and releasing our struggles to Him.

· refusing to escape into the old patterns, habits, and attitudes that continue to distract us. and add to the destruction of our lives.

· no longer saying, "I can handle this myself."

· submitting to God's way of doing things even when we don't understand.

· getting past our pain and fear and clinging to our hope in God and His love for us.

· setting aside our human understanding and becoming childlike, and acknowledging we have no answers that work.

Surrender allows you to grow as you submit to God's authority. In order to submit, you must trust that God has good things for you and that His plans and purposes far outweigh what you bring to the table. There are times in our lives when it is very tough to believe that God has good plans in store. When I (Steve) discovered my marriage would end in divorce, it caused a huge faith crisis for me. Surely God would want to spare me the embarrassment and humiliation of being divorced in front of radio listeners, book readers, friends, and family, wouldn't He? What could ever come out of all of this that would be good? Though I never doubted Jesus was the only way to heaven, I did start to doubt if God really was involved with my life on this side of heaven. I was in deep pain and didn't know if I could trust God to be personally involved with me.

Daily surrender was a daily battle. I felt the need to control based on the absence of His "felt" concern. So I set out in the beginning to do the best I could under my own power. Fortunately that plan did not last long. I began to see God at work and trusted that His love was still there for me in the midst of my failed marriage. Through this pain I came to realize that much of my life was not surrendered. As a result of that crisis, I came to a fresher seeking of the true and living God, complete with a new desire for intimacy with Him. The divorce was just the excuse God used to bring me to my knees and to get to know Him once again.

In my own life, I (Dr. Linda) struggled with this concept after my

The difference between surrender and control looks like this:

SURRENDER	CONTROL
God is the Master of the universe.	I can master all things.
God's perspective is higher than mine.	What I feel is all that is important.
My circumstances are part of God's eternal perspective.	If God is God, my circumstances must be changed now.
I must allow God's plans to open up before me.	My plans are all that matter. I demand immediate results.
I am not alone and will never be.	If there is a God, He is not a part of my life, and I alone can change my reality.
I accept life knowing that all things will work together for my good.	I blame God when life doesn't go the way I think it should.

oldest brother was killed. I falsely believed that God could not be trusted because He didn't protect my family and prevent this tragedy from happening. At a time of great loss, I believed a lie—that God could not be trusted. So why would I submit to such an authority?

The lie became so ingrained that a few years later, I refused to put the words "submit" and "obey" in my wedding vows. I loved my husband-to-be, but would I submit to his authority and trust that he had good things for me? No way. My husband, like God, could not be trusted; both had the potential to hurt me. My belief wasn't based on any reality—I just wasn't about to give control to anyone for fear of being hurt. Disappointed with God, I thought I could prevent bad things from happening. I figured the more I took charge of my life, the less chance I had to be hurt again. You can guess how well this strategy worked!

The years of heartache this type of thinking caused could have been avoided if I had recognized the lie under which I was operating. I had an inaccurate view of God based on my traumatic experience of loss. As a young adult, this prevented me from submitting my life to God's greater purposes, a step that could have saved me much grief. Be assured that it is never too late to abandon yourself to God's power and authority. He can redeem lost time and work His purposes in your life. This has been true in my own life. And when you release yourself from self-effort and striving, a huge burden is lifted.

Thus, your first step to "lose it for life" is to acknowledge your incredible need for God to take the reigns. If you don't do this, you are doomed to continue to try every new diet or scheme that offers you false hope and false security. But if you can grasp this concept of surrender and implement it, you can be free from your obsessions and find a new life you never dreamed could be so great. But understand, before you can have that life, you must surrender the one you have.

Surrender acknowledges God's existence and is the first act of faith that will begin your transformation. If you want to get off the weight-loss roller coaster, then surrender to God's way of doing things. Acknowledge that He is in the driver's seat and you are along for the ride. Your way hasn't worked and His grace is sufficient. His power will be made perfect in your weakness. Surrender leads to healing and the promise God gave us in Jeremiah 29:14: "'I will be found by you,' declares the LORD, 'and will bring you back from captivity.'"

> *Dear Lord,*
>
> *I surrender my life to you. Open my eyes to the truth of who You are and what You desire to do in my life. Show me specific areas of my life that need to be surrendered to You. Help me to seek You with my whole heart so that You may reveal yourself to me and I may find You. Lead me to those who will help me on this journey. Fill me with Your love and give me what I need to choose Your way and*

not mine. I trust You enough to surrender my life to You without condition or demands. I trust You to love me, to take care of me, and to never leave me. Please help me to realize whenever I am trying to control You, so that I can surrender to You and let You control my life. Amen.

Meet Grace, a Needed Friend

Once the decision to surrender all to Christ is made, transformation begins. During the process, you'll be introduced to a friend who can really help. Perhaps you've never met this person, or maybe you have but never took the time to get to know him.

Lose it for lifer—Meet GRACE.

Grace is divine, a gift from God to you. He offers new life based on nothing you have to offer. There is no way to earn His affections or coax His love for you. He already delights in you and befriends you. The fact that you are overweight and feel like such a failure doesn't impact Him. When you fail, He says, "Not to worry. I am with you and we can start afresh. Lean on Me, not on your own strength. I am strong when you are weak. I have a plan and purpose for your life that I'm dying to reveal."

This guy seems too good to be true, you think. *Perhaps there is a catch.* But as you become more acquainted with Grace, you see He is authentic. There is no pretending. He is compassionate and He cares deeply. And He has the capacity to be intimately involved in your life. His friendship and promises are mind-boggling. People sing and talk about Him and describe Him as "amazing." Apparently He has quite the reputation for being "The Man," despite His feminine name. One reason relates to His astounding ability to see sin, not excuse it, but love anyway. He hangs out with the failed, the most desperate, and the most defeated. He walks along, holding their hands and pours out healing salve, mercy, and hope. Grace is shocking in the way He upholds the unlovely.

And He knows your critical thought, *If I really wanted to lose weight, I would!* But He responds with such confidence: "I know what you want . . . but don't worry about your life, what you will eat or what you will drink; or about your body, what you will put on." Grace's passion for you is so powerful that it overcomes your fears.

Grace understands the angst involved in doing what you hate— overeating, dieting, gaining momentary control, and overeating again— and says, "Hey, you can't do this on your own. There are healthy ways to eat, but you won't make it with self-imposed rules. I am here to help you change your life, not just your eating. Without Me, it's pretty hopeless—a sort of grit-your-teeth-and-hang-on existence. You need Me in your life. Take Me on your journey."

According to our reports, Grace was recently spotted having lunch with a bunch of overeaters. Many were downright obese and had given up hope for any future joy. But Grace didn't seem to be embarrassed. His kindness was so refreshing. And His eyes . . . well, all you could see was compassion.

*Patiently He listened as the group recited their various individual struggles from a week of dieting. Then He gently spoke. "Wow, all you talk about are standards and rules—Never mess up the diet. Don't touch chocolate again. Condemn yourself if you fall into temptation. And these rules seem to be written in stone! You guys need a break. These laws and rules are **guidelines** for eating, but they are impossible to keep all the time. Aren't you human? It's OK to mess up. Just acknowledge when you do, turn from it, and start over.*

"With My help, you can keep moving toward the goal. However, remind yourself about Me. I'm going to be here every day. Without Me, your heart will condemn you. But I won't withhold any good thing from you if you walk uprightly."

Stunned, the group sat in silence. One brave woman spoke. "I've

> *never met anyone like You. My friends and co-workers judge me because of the way I look. They say I am fat and lazy and will never be promoted. You say You have good things for me? By the way, did You notice I weigh 280 pounds?"*
>
> *"I noticed," Grace replied. "But I fail to see how that relates to My offer. Apparently you don't get it. I'm not basing My care for you on anything you do or on how you appear. I would love your devotion in return, but it isn't contingent on Me loving you."*
>
> *"OK!" an angry man yelled back. "How much is this going to cost us? What's the bottom line?"*
>
> *"The cost has already been paid. You were bought with a price. What I have, I give freely. There is no additional cost. It was a one-time deal. Paid in full. Sealed."*

Who is this marvelous friend? John 1:17 reveals Him: "For the law was given through Moses; grace and truth came through Jesus Christ." The grace of God is revealed through the divine person and work of Jesus Christ. He both embodied grace and benefited from God's grace. By His death and resurrection on the cross, Christ brought salvation to each of us and restored our broken relationship with God. The Holy Spirit, called the Spirit of grace (Hebrews 10:29 NKJV), is the one who binds Christ to us so that we can receive forgiveness, adoption, and new life.

Grace requires faith. We must trust in the mercy of God and realize His favor on us even though it is undeserved. This unmerited favor is a free gift given by our affectionate heavenly Father. As we "lose it for life," we must remember that God's grace abounds in our lives. He is for us, not against us. He cheers us on to victory, and He uses others to pour out that grace in our lives as well.

If you find you are beating yourself up all the time, saying to yourself things you would never say to someone else, then you have GD (Grace Deficiency). If you think you are so bad no one can love you, you have GD. If you judge yourself based solely on your weight, you have GD. Thankfully, this misery-inducing disease has a cure! God's extravagant grace is what heals it. Give yourself a Grace transfusion through the reading of God's Word, communing with His people, and utilizing a new vocabulary for your self-talk. It is time you started treating yourself the way God treats you . . . with Grace!

Counting the Costs

Grace is an amazing gift from God. But it does not entitle us to a free ride with no effort on our part. Losing weight and keeping it off under a shower of God's grace still requires small amounts of sacrifice and pain. It is going to cost you more than just developing some good intentions, which people usually have when they approach weight loss. However, in our experience, few people really think through all the ramifications of their weight loss decisions up front. We believe this has something to do with why so many people fail to keep weight off and give up the battle so quickly. But we are not interested in witnessing your failure, so read on!

Do you recall the story of Jesus and the rich young ruler found in Matthew 19:16-22? The story illustrates the importance of counting the cost before you make a decision. In the story, there is a rich young ruler who approaches Jesus and says, "Good Teacher, what good thing shall I do that I may have eternal life?" Jesus answers by stating five of the ten commandments and adds that the man should love his neighbor as himself. The young man acknowledges having done all these things and further asks, "What do I still lack?" to which Jesus replies, "Sell what you have and give to the poor . . . come, follow Me" (NKJV). Suddenly, the rich young ruler feels the weight of what he is being asked to do. It's one thing to be good and keep the commandments, another to give up what he already has (or thinks he has). You see, his wealth really wasn't his problem. A divided heart was the issue. He wasn't sure he could give up his security for the promise of eternal life. Sadly, he did not follow Jesus because he concluded that the cost was too great.

Do you see the parallels? Whenever you make a decision to change things about your life, there are costs to consider, and your heart cannot be divided as you decide. Perhaps you are more comfortable with dieting than you even know. You try to be good—you even keep all the dieting commandments (Thou shall eat only low-fat foods. Thou shall have no chocolate, etc.) and also wonder, "What do I still lack?" Notice the specific answer Jesus gives. There is no question what is required— total surrender.

Note that Jesus not only gave a specific answer but also addressed the heart condition of the young man. He was looking for a heart sold out to Him. In order to live a life undefined by your weight, your heart condition is critical. Your weight isn't the root problem. Oh, it's tipping the scales too high or causing you distress; we understand this. But there is more to losing and keeping weight off than meets the eye. The good outcome you desire requires changes of behavior, thinking, and the heart.

Even though this might be difficult to accept, it should be a source of hope for you. Other diet books have not helped you because they have addressed only one aspect of the problem—what is going into your mouth. And you have likely proven that for a specific amount of time you can change what you eat. But it is a change of the heart that sustains change in terms of what you eat and fuels a desire to find the weight that is right for you. Heart change is not easy work, but it is easier than staying where you are and experiencing the same frustrations and failures.

We want to be clear from the start: There are no magic pills to offer you. We have no gimmicks, no quick fixes; there are no melt-away-the-pounds creams or cookies that fuel your metabolism into burning like the blazing sun. But there is a path to follow that will transform your life and bring about a stronger, clearer sense of you, as well as healing, renewed thoughts, and meaningful connections.

So let's begin to identify the possible changes you could encounter. Think about these *before* the going gets tough so you can remain tough and keep going. We believe the benefits of a changed life are worth the costs, but you must decide for yourself by counting the costs before committing.

Overeating serves a purpose. This purpose may not be healthy, desired, or even in your awareness, but it is there. Try to think about what it would mean to lose that extra weight and keep it off for life. It's important to be realistic when seeking answers for why you want to be thin. Think about what your life would be like if you didn't spend so much time and energy with food. For example, you might have extra time to fill. With what would you fill it? Would you feel more anxious if your life didn't revolve around food? Most people do experience anxiety when they stop using food to cope with stress because they have to learn new ways to cope. Change, even when desired and positive, can be stressful.

One important question to ask is this: "Will I be confronted with issues in my life I have worked hard to avoid?" For example, maybe you are secretly angry over your husband's request for a divorce and you have stuffed those feelings away by eating. If you stop using food to dull the pain, those feelings of hurt may surface. And though you can learn to tolerate this, it won't be pleasant. You will have to learn to manage those feelings and deal with them directly.

In Order to Lose Weight and Keep It Off, I Might Be Changing . . .

There are a multitude of changes that occur when people try to give up a lifetime of food and weight problems. Although some of these may apply to you, others will not. And there may be personal changes that will occur that only you know about, so we've left a blank line. Take a moment to read through this list and decide if any of these apply to you. And feel free to jot down others that come to mind.

1. **A comfortable habit and way of life.** Eating is what I do when I am happy, comfortable, and feeling good. It's social and a way of life. Go to a movie without a bucket of popcorn? No way.

2. **My best and most acceptable form of distraction.** For example, it's easier to think about the next meal, binge, or snack than the way my boss just treated me on the phone.

3. **A meaningful expression of love.** Food and love are closely associated. Cooking and eating high-calorie foods may be a way you give and receive love.

4. **A way to satisfy needs.** Do I eat as a response to a felt need? Even though the food doesn't satisfy that need, I eat *as if* it does.

5. **Protection from my own sexual impulses.** To lose weight means feeling more attractive. Can I control those impulses related to feeling more sexual and satisfied with my body when I lose weight?

6. **Protection from the sexual advances of others.** If I was raped or sexually abused when I was thin, I might believe that my weight has served as protection against further abuse. If I lose weight, will I feel more vulnerable? Am I ready and willing to face this?

7. **A strategy to keep an intimate other at bay.** When I feel unattractive and don't like my body, I have an excuse to avoid intimacy (especially with my spouse). Am I ready to confront ALL the issues that come with building intimacy?

8. **A cover-up for fears, including failure.** The reason I'm not married, the reason I lost my job, the reason I can't make friends . . . is because I'm fat. Could there be other reasons?

9. **A way to control my life with false structure.** When I feel out of control, eating can be a way to structure my life.

10. **A major coping mechanism for life's stresses.** A general pattern has developed. When I am stressed, I eat. Yes, STRESSED is DESSERTS spelled backwards!

11. **My tried-and-true way to deal with boredom.** Boredom can be relieved by adding a little spice to life—with extra pasta, a little more sauce. When I open the refrigerator I find something interesting.

12. **My best friend.** Food never lets me down. I can always depend on it being there and making me feel good for the moment.

13. **My most dependable way to experience pleasure.** There is pleasure in eating, in taste, in texture. And hey, according to our culture, I deserve to feel pleasure (and lots of it!) whenever I want it.

14. **The best or most acceptable numbing device used for emotional pain and anger.** Eating really works to distract me from emotional pain and anger. I don't have to think or feel—just eat.

15. **Protection from rejection.** My layers of fat protect me from possible rejection. I don't have to date, ski, go to the beach, or assert myself—after all, I am fat.

16. **Fantasy versus reality.** If I was thinner . . . ahhh, let me dream of the good life and fantasize about all my problems melting away with the fat. There's no need for reality to interfere.

17. **A way of thinking that reinforces those feelings of not being good enough.** When I am overweight, I can continue to find reasons why people won't like me. They won't look beyond my weight to really get to know me. Without the weight, well . . . I don't want to think there could be other things about me they might not like.

18. **Waiting for the future to avoid the NOW.** When I am down to a size 14, *then* I'll visit my relatives. When I fit into that dress, *then* I'll talk to men. The list for future action just grows with the weight gain.

19. **Pretending I have no problems.** "Hey, I'm the life of the party, easygoing, and can get along with anyone. Everyone likes me." It's true. I never assert myself and instead pretend I don't have needs. I use food to cover hurtful feelings. My life is dedicated to helping others. It's selfish to think about me.

20. _____

What Works and What Doesn't

Finally, you may be wondering if this program will be any different from your past efforts to lose weight. Perhaps you've yo-yo dieted or lost a great deal of weight only to put it all back on with a few additional pounds. If so, consider the following ten pros and cons of why other programs fail, as well as the alternatives offered by Lose It For Life.

When making any decision, weigh the pros and cons related to change. If you desire in your heart to do this, God will empower you to deal with the hurdles along the way—that is His promise. Through His Spirit, as you surrender to Him and accept His grace, He will transform you to His image. He is your help and source of strength. Invite Him to walk alongside of you. His desire is to change your entire life, both physically and spiritually.

Surrender is one of the transforming keys that begins the process of losing the weight for life. In order to give up control and trust God, get to know Him better. Read what the Word says about who He is and what He promises He will do for you. "Taste and see that the LORD is good; blessed is the man [or woman] who takes refuge in him" (Psalm 34:8, emphasis added). Around the corner is true freedom—much more than just weight loss! The decision is yours.

OTHER DIETS & PROGRAMS	LOSE IT FOR LIFE
Unrealistic expectations. People are often disappointed by the reality that weight loss doesn't fix other problems.	**Realistic expectations.** This especially applies to losing weight slowly and sensibly. Other areas of your life may require examination.
Weight loss motivated by appearance. Improving health is more important than becoming thin.	**Changing the focus to health and lifestyle.** This is a lifelong journey with a focus away from weight to that of improved health.
Eating low-fat but still gaining weight. We've developed a diet mentality in which we think low-fat means weight loss. Actually you can eat low-fat food in large quantities and still gain weight.	**Cutting back on high glycemic foods** (sugar and refined carbohydrates). For long-term success, feeling more energetic, and eating healthier, this helps.
Physical activity was not increased. Long term, you won't maintain weight loss if you don't increase your physical movement.	**Increased exercise and movement.** In most cases, 30-60 minutes of exercise, five to seven days a week keeps the weight off. The more active you are the better.
All the issues involved in overeating are not addressed. Too many programs focus only on weight loss. Weight loss must address all aspects of your life.	**Resolving emotional issues.** Filling emotional and relational needs with food doesn't work.
Health issues that contributed to weight gain were ignored. You need to know what is causing your weight gain.	**Encouraging Self-Monitoring.** This means weighing regularly, being aware of how your clothes fit, and looking at your body. In addition, medical monitoring may be necessary if you have health issues.
Disconnecting the spiritual and the body. Your spiritual life is directly related to your physical life. Your body is the temple of the Holy Spirit. Both need to be fed.	**Support a vibrant spiritual life.** We are all in desperate need of mind renewal and allowing God to give us hearts of flesh in exchange for our hearts of stone.
Nutritional plan didn't work. In the world of food and eating, one size does not fit all. You have to develop eating habits that work for you, are balanced, and provide proper nutrition.	**Eating at regular times in order to maximize your body's metabolism.** The idea of skipping meals doesn't work. It sets you up to overeat, crave foods, and slows down your metabolism.
Lack of support. Research shows that social support helps sustain weight loss efforts and maintenance. Spouses are especially important because they can unknowingly sabotage your efforts.	**Connection and Support.** Research is clear that support is needed. You will need to build community with people who will support and help you.
Not patient enough. Any lifestyle change takes time to incorporate. Remember, slow and steady wins the race. Quick weight loss methods usually fail long term.	**Balance and moderation.** It will become your mantra: "There are no forbidden foods." By not feeling deprived, you will stick with the plan and lose it for life!

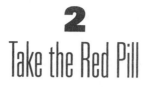

2
Take the Red Pill

*O LORD, you have examined my heart
and know everything about me.*
— PSALM 139:1 NLT

If you saw *The Matrix*, you'll understand this next challenge. It involves just one question: Will you take the red pill? For those of you who didn't see the movie or prefer not to, here's the context. In *The Matrix*, a computer hacker named Neo lives a rather ordinary life in what he thinks is the year 1999. Morpheus, a rebel warrior, contacts Neo and explains to him that his reality is in fact false. The truth is that it is 200 years later, artificial intelligence runs the world, and humans are living in a complex system in which they are placated and used for fuel to run the machines that have very nearly taken over the world. Neo, fresh with this revelation, is confronted with a life-altering choice: He can take the blue pill, wake up the next morning remembering nothing of this meeting and go on living in his false world, or he can take the red pill. If he swallows the red pill, he'll see life as it really is (and save the world, of course!).

Think of yourself as Neo. We (Morpheus) are confronting you with a life-altering choice. Do you want to continue to live in the false world of dieting, where emotional pain is numbed, health risks are ignored, and false promises are made? Or do you want to take the red pill, as it were, and see the reality of a world in which food and eating don't dominate or take over your life? If you accept this challenge, you will have to face moments of pain from the past you might prefer be left alone, deal with relationship difficulties, and make changes in possibly all aspects of your lifestyle. As you consider, ask yourself what would happen if your body was how you wanted it to be and food no longer ruled your day.

Lose It For Life is a program that can make this happen. Change is possible, and the support and insight in this book can help you be successful as you commit to getting healthy and staying on track. One step at a time, through making decisions and evaluating your needs, you will find the answers you need.

If you do choose the red pill, you won't be saving the whole world, but your whole world will change as you reclaim your sanity and health!

Accepting Reality

Once you fully surrender the weight loss battle to God, you must open your eyes to reality and stop lying to yourself or making excuses. This is a vital step in the process. Incredible insight concerning Truth is offered by Dostoevsky in his novel *The Brothers Karamazov:*

> The important thing is to stop lying to yourself. A man who lies to himself, and believes his lies, becomes unable to recognize the truth, either in himself or anyone else, and he ends up losing respect for himself as well as others. When he has no respect for anyone, he can no longer love and, in order to divert himself, having no love in him, he yields to his impulses, indulges in the lowest forms of pleasure, and behaves in the end like an animal, in satisfying his vices. And it all comes from lying—lying to others and to yourself.

In order to lose weight for life, you have to face reality or you end up lying to yourself and others. Tough questions must be asked and answered:

· What is my part in gaining this weight?

· How do I respond to difficulty?

· What unmet needs do I have that I try to meet through food?

· When life gets tough, do I get going or start eating?

· Am I hung up on "why" my life feels so out of control?

· Am I disconnected from others?

· Do I live in denial, refusing to acknowledge my weight problem and the impact it has on my life?

The words of Jesus in John 16:33 provide truth and hope. Jesus tells His disciples, "These things I have spoken to you, that in Me you may have peace. In the world you will have tribulation; but be of good cheer, I have overcome the world" (NKJV).

Jesus doesn't lie to us. As the Son of God, He is incapable of lying. He tells us that difficulty and suffering will be part of life—He wants us to know reality. And this is the reason we can trust Christ: He is the Truth and He speaks truth. Jesus offers hope. He has overcome the world! During His life on earth, He overcame Satan's temptation. On the cross, He overcame the power of sin by becoming sin. And through His death and resurrection, He broke the power of death. He is our hope no matter what difficulty we face. "I am the way, the truth, and the life. No one comes to the Father except through me," He declares (John 14:6 NKJV). "And you shall know the truth, and the truth shall make you free" (John 8:32 NKJV). Acceptance involves first realizing the full depth of your problem . . . which means taking the red pill and seeing life as it really is.

So often it is easier to replace these realities with lies of our own making. We tell ourselves there really is nothing we can do; that it isn't our fault we got so heavy; or that to face the reality will mean facing pain, which is potentially worse than letting ourselves go and merely surviving through life. Or we assume that if God wanted to, He would take this burden from us. He would take away this pain if it were His will.

Your overweight body is a symptom of an under-developed soul.

No one else caused your problem, and no one else is going to fix it for you.

When you decide to change, it is going to be painful.

No one can walk through that pain but you, and you must walk through it.

All are very tempting lies to hold onto, but when we reach that point of acceptance, the lies start to peel away. Reality is no longer denied and the truth comes out: Being overweight is not about the past, or food, or even the temporary relief and comfort found in food. *It is about right now and what you choose to do about it.* A weight problem either continues to get worse or gets better with the next choice made. Take note—no matter what path was chosen before, choosing differently *now* is the key to where this program begins.

Break Through Your Denial

All of us struggle with blind spots in our lives, and to some degree we all live in the company of denial and self-deception. But rather than confront our area(s) of struggle and pain, we often point to others and focus on them or find alternatives to distract and anesthetize ourselves from what really needs to be faced.

Acceptance is being willing to lift the curtain of denial and look at the big lie of your life. Breaking through denial means being aware of your struggle and pain and consciously confronting the behaviors and patterns that have deterred you from God's best. Only with God's help and a supportive, healing community can the blinders be removed.

Deception and denial give way to seeing yourself as you really are—trapped in your patterns, paralyzed by fear, and making choices that produce short-term results rather than long-term change. God is patient, loving, and able "to do far more than we would ever dare to ask or even dream of—infinitely beyond our highest prayers, desires, thoughts, or hopes" (Ephesians 3:20 TLB). Take a moment and examine your heart. How have you avoided reality? See if any of these actions play a role in how you avoid the truth:

- You avoid prayer, times of silence and looking at your situation, honest conversations that touch a sensitive area of your life, or people who can speak into your life and encourage you on your journey.
- You minimize or rationalize your behavior.
- You constantly criticize others.
- You are confused as to why others react to you and what you say or do.
- You find yourself lying repeatedly.

If you are willing to confront the reality of your overeating, these positive signs will be evident:

- You focus on what you can do to change rather than on what you want others to do to make you feel better.
- You humble yourself in order to confront who you really are.
- You look for what really causes the conflicts you experience.
- You honestly face your past pain and failures head on.
- You stop blaming others for your difficulties.
- You seek, receive, and apply God's wisdom to your situation.
- You look at what you've done in the light of God's mercy and grace—not judgment or condemnation.
- You accept that you are unable to help yourself without God's help.
- You can name your character defects and mistakes rather than deny them.

By being honest you can move out of the past and into the reality of the present. Only when you face the truth can God teach you to resolve your problems rather than reproduce them within relationships with family and close friends. Are you ready to take the red pill? It's a big dose of reality, but with God's help and the help of others, you can take it.

Dear Lord,

Open my eyes to see the truth about You and myself. Show me the things that need to be changed. Put me on the right path that I may walk in Your truth. Amen.

Letting Go of Excuses

Making excuses is perhaps the most common way to justify overeating—and deal with failure. With a good excuse, guilt and anxiety about overeating dissipate. But the sad reality is that making excuses to feel better about overeating actually fosters continued overeating by simply lessening the momentary anxiety—which means making excuses becomes part of a vicious cycle of overeating again and again.

For example, it's late at night. You are watching TV and you start thinking about ice cream because you've just seen a tantalizing commercial. Anxiety begins to mount as you try to decide if you should eat the ice cream sitting in your freezer . . . or say no. You aren't thinking about the fact that you are *not* hungry. The ice cream just looks so good—it would be a terrific treat right now . . . and it's calling to you from the freezer . . . and you've had a long and exhausting day. All of these are excuses that hide the truth: *You are not hungry.* But the excuses come so easily, so smoothly, it has become your habit to just ignore the truth when it comes to overeating. Excuses take the focus off of the long-term consequences.

Certainly you don't want to think about the long-term effects of overeating right now. And the longer you postpone eating the ice cream, the greater your anxiety becomes. *Should I eat or shouldn't I?* Eventually you become so uncomfortable over this dilemma that you get up, walk to the kitchen, and serve yourself a scoop of ice cream.

Then you think, *There isn't that much ice cream left in the carton. I'll finish it off and won't buy anymore. I'll start dieting tomorrow when it's all gone.* As you begin to overeat, the momentary anxiety disappears. The ice cream tastes great, or at least you think it did—you ate it so fast, you really didn't taste it. Now it's late, and now you are really tired. Feeling uncomfortably full, you go to bed.

Excuses prompted you to avoid the reality that you weren't hungry. Sound familiar? Happily, there is an alternative, but the first step is to see excuses for what they really are.

Think It Through—Delay Gratification

When you ate the ice cream, you gave in—you bowed under pressure to the moment (and the anxiety) without thinking about the long-term consequences. You are an advertiser's dream TV viewer! Immediate gratification is the message advertisers sell. Their job is to persuade you to be impulsive, to give in to temptation.

To lose weight and keep it off requires you to delay momentary gratification and think with a long-term perspective—to engage in the reality of your decisions. Advertisers hope you won't think that hard. They would prefer that you live in the moment and give in to the immediate pleasures they are selling. However, when you are tempted, think about the impact of this one choice on your life. Taking the earlier example, ask yourself questions like these:

· How will I feel after I eat this?
· How will I feel in thirty minutes?
· How will I feel about this tomorrow morning?

· Will I beat myself up over this choice?

You get the idea. To delay an urge to overeat, don't rationalize what you are doing. Think about the long-term consequences and learn to tolerate your anxious feelings, which generally will pass after only a short time. Tell yourself it's normal to feel anxious when making a decision. Take a few deep breaths and relax your body; the urge will likely subside within twenty minutes or so.

Or wait for that anxious feeling to go away by distracting yourself with something else. Turn off the TV, pull out a book, call a friend, take a walk, go to the bathroom (people tend not to eat in the bathroom), get in the car and go for a drive, attend a meeting, or just go to bed. Whatever you do, don't stare at the refrigerator and try to exercise willpower.

These strategies work for overeating and other impulsive behavior as well. And sometimes the best strategy is to avoid any tempting situation altogether. Late-night TV viewing may be a trigger for you to overeat. If so, don't watch late-night TV! Instead, do something different: play a game, read, pray for your family, or do a Bible study.

If you do decide to give in to the immediate pleasure of eating, take *one* scoop of ice cream and no more. Eat it slowly and enjoy every bite. You won't gain a pound from one small scoop, but eating the entire carton will certainly do some damage. The next day, be sure that you go to the store and replace that high-fat, high-carb, high-sugar ice cream with a no-sugar-added substitute. Make your freezer safe for the next time you just can't resist or are unwilling to delay gratification.

Delaying gratification is a process that involves self-control, an area we often feel we lack in. According to Galatians 5:22-23, self-control is a fruit of the Spirit. This fruit is an attribute of those who walk in the Spirit. As we grow in the Lord, we become more like Him.

Just as fruit begins with a seed, so too does a fruitful spiritual life. Both need nourishment to thrive. We need to read the Word of God and let it soak very deep in our hearts. The more we desire to please God in all we do, the more obedient we become. Obedience produces self-discipline, which gives way to self-control. We are not talking about control born of self-effort, but self-control born of the Spirit working in us.

The enemy of our souls wants to discourage us from ever thinking we could have a supernatural self-control. Satan even tested Jesus in the wilderness. This fallen angel came to Jesus when He was physically weak, hungry, and tired from fasting. Just think, the first wilderness temptation involved food, as did the original temptation with Adam and Eve!

Satan, knowing the toll of hunger on Jesus' earthly body, suggested a shortcut—an immediate gratification. However, the biblical account begins with an important fact. *The Spirit* led Jesus into the wilderness. Don't miss the importance of this—being led by the Spirit is what we all need in order to overcome our weaknesses.

And Jesus' defense against succumbing to immediate gratification was to quote the Word to His enemy. The Living Word quoted the Word. This is your model for overcoming. As you soak yourself in the Word, you nourish your spiritual life. The seed bears fruit—in this case, self-control. Be ready for times of testing. Nourish yourself with plenty of time in the Word and allow your life to bear the fruit of the Spirit

Responsibility—the Balance to Surrender

Another key element of a life no longer controlled by appetite or weight is a newfound sense of responsibility. We must refuse to blame anyone else for the extra weight and acknowledge that we are responsible, yet we can't fix this on our own power. This is the balance of surrendering to God: We allow God to do what we cannot do, but we do what we can.

Responsibility involves the treatment of old wounds that may be triggering your overeating. It also requires making strong decisions and changes in your life. Hurts that drive you to inappropriate behaviors and destructive habits are hurts that you may never have fully worked through. Diverting yourself from problems or anesthetizing your emotions with food, hurtful people, or activities may be a common pattern in your life.

The Steps of Accepting Responsibility

1. Facing problems rather than escaping them, including bearing the full responsibility of misconduct.

2. Taking time to grieve the loss and experience pain—"Blessed are those who mourn, for they will be comforted" (Matthew 5:4).

3. Reaching out to Christ, who suffered Himself and understands our hurt.

4. Accepting the hope that God's plans for us are good and loving—we must purposefully look beyond the loss to God's deeper purposes.

5. Refusing to allow anything from the past to serve as an excuse for lack of growth, character, or development, including living in the role of victim.

In our world, it's easy to take on the role of victim and live a life of victimization. Yet, as horrendous as your past problems and abuse may have been, when you own them as part of you, you learn to see them as purposeful, deepening, and integral to your development of godly character.

It takes courage to walk through this pain, but God can provide the strength and support to truly overcome past hurts and, ultimately, to use them for His glory. As the psalmist David wrote, "It was good for me to be afflicted so that I might learn your decrees" (Psalm 119:71).

Avoiding pain and problems is a natural human response. Most people feel they have "suffered enough" and have no desire to feel overwhelmed by sorrowful emotions. But grief is a necessary process of this earthly life, because we all fail, suffer, and deal with loss. It is important to note that experiencing grief over our failures and losses connects us to God's grace. Saint Augustine affirmed this when he said, "In my deepest wound I saw your glory and it dazzled me." It is not pleasant, but it is necessary. We must experience (or grieve) the pain we feel today so we will not be driven by it in the future. Too often we point to our past pain as an excuse and miss the fact that it very definitely *is* part of God's plan for us. It is so easy to blame others for everything that has gone wrong. When we don't accept responsibility, we live in a victimized state and blame others for our problems. For the overeater, food will continue to be used to deaden pain and numb reality.

Prayer for Accepting Responsibility

Dear Lord,

I realize You have given me life and that living is my responsibility. Lord, I want to accept responsibility for my whole life. I know You want my life to be fruitful, but sin and tragedy have infected my life—both by my hand and the hands of others. Help me to accept responsibility to remove these weeds that have been sown in me. Lord, I confess that sometimes I blame others for my own disobedience to You. I now accept responsibility for these things. Please forgive me and fully restore the relationship between us. Amen.

Examine Your Motivation

When you give up your excuses, pray a prayer of acceptance and responsibility, and then examine your motivation for wanting to lose weight. If your main motivation is to be thin so you can do all the things you never could do before, or to be the person you were never allowed to be and have all your dreams come true, it's time to reevaluate (definitely take the red pill!).

Research tells us that people become more successful at long-term weight loss when their motivation is to become *healthier,* not thinner. This change in attitude or motivation is essential. Improving your health involves lifestyle changes that we will delineate in this book. To be thin, you have to lose the weight. And we know you can do that. Many of you have done so, *over and over.* To lose it for life, you have to take a more comprehensive approach. All the areas involved with over-eating must be addressed.

Write It Down

Perhaps you are frustrated because it seems like you've been dieting forever and haven't lost a pound. We can relate. My college "cottage cheese diet" caused me (Dr. Linda) to gain fifteen pounds my freshman year. Here's what I did. I skipped breakfast every day (and slept instead), ate cottage cheese and fruit for lunch, and then ate a regular dinner. As I stared at my little bowl of white mealy curds every lunchtime, I believed I was making the ultimate sacrifice to lose weight. (For the record, I don't believe cottage cheese is real food!) But I ate it religiously and sincerely thought the pounds would fall off.

What I failed to take into account was a small but important fact. Snack machines were placed in the dorms and right next to the room where I studied. In addition to my meals, I was also ingesting late-night fruit pies from those machines. Oh yes, and those cinnamon buns . . . and maybe a few Doritos™ too. And when the chocolate was passed around the study room, I broke off my share of the bar. All those extra calories that didn't "count" because they weren't part of my meals added up to quite a shocking number! No wonder I didn't lose weight.

Maybe it seems like you eat very little. Or you think you can't lose weight on a 1,200-calorie diet because of metabolic problems or heredity issues. Yet in truth, very few people have metabolic disorders or genetic factors that cause them to be overweight. Because so many people reported eating small amounts of food and gaining weight, researchers studied this. What they found was that people grossly underestimated what they ate in a day, and they also exercised less than they thought.[7] It wasn't that people were intentionally lying about what they ate. They just forgot about moments in the day when they grabbed a handful of M&Ms™ or tasted spoonfuls of chili while preparing dinner. A little here and a little there really adds up.

Perhaps the largest number of "hidden" calories and carbs are consumed in the most unnoticed way—in what you drink. Soft drinks and hard liquor and everything in between fill us up with calories that often go unaccounted. Consider this reality: If in a single day you consumed a twelve-ounce mocha, two glasses of orange juice, two glasses of milk, a can of regular soda, and a twelve-ounce bottle of beer, you added nearly a thousand calories to the total number of calories you consumed in actual food!

Studies show that people who record what they eat lose more weight and keep it off compared to those who don't. In fact, the more days a person keeps a food journal, the greater the weight loss.[8] So, based on studies and our personal experience, keeping a food journal is important. Begin by writing down everything you eat in a day for a week or two. It sounds tedious, but recording this data will provide you with a greater awareness of what you are eating. A food journal will also pinpoint eating patterns—when you eat, how much, how often, the amount of what you eat, etc. This information will later be used to make changes. Here is a sample of a simple food journal. (See Appendix A for a blank copy. The *Lose It For Life Interactive Journal Planner* is another resource and is available from the loseitforlife.com Web site.)

It was eye-opening for Jane to track her food intake every day for two weeks. You can see just by glancing at this first day of Jane's food journal, as she did, how the calories added up and how many empty-calorie, non-nutritional foods she consumed. Fruits, vegetables, and protein were lacking in her food choices. In addition, she often ate on the run while doing errands in her car, with only one meal being eaten at her kitchen table. There were times she ate when she wasn't even hungry, as well as instances where the meal included multiple servings

Food Journal

Name: Jane Doe

Date: Wednesday, May 18

When I ate	Where I ate	What I ate	How much I ate	Was I hungry?
Breakfast 8 a.m.	Kitchen table	Jelly donuts	3	Yes
		Coffee with cream and sugar	3 cups, 3 tbsp., 2 tbsp.	Yes
		Orange juice	1 cup	Yes
10 a.m.	Desk at work	Pop Tart™	2	Yes
11 a.m.	Car	Bag of chips	12 oz.	No
Lunch 12 p.m.	Mall Plaza	Pizza	3 slices	Yes
		Coke™	1 24-oz. Cup	Yes
	Car	Heath™ Ice Cream	1 Klondike™ bar	No
2 p.m.	Desk	Cupcakes	2	No
4 p.m.	Car	French fries	1 large	No
		Coke™	12 oz.	No
		Burger	1 regular	No
Dinner 6 p.m.	In front of TV	Lasagna	2 large helpings	Yes
		Salad with dressing	1 bowl with ¼ cup bleu cheese	Yes
		Bread sticks	3	No
		Dr. Pepper™	2 8-oz. Cans	Yes
		Cheesecake	1 large slice	No
		Coffee with cream and sugar	2 cups, 3 tbsp., 2 tbsp.	No
8:30 p.m.	Movie	Buttered popcorn	Large bag	No
		Sprite™	2 8-oz. Glasses	No

or large-size items. Without the help of a dictitian, Jane could see she had to make changes—thanks to the food journal, which provided her an objective view of her eating patterns.

Identify Your Eating Patterns

There are basically three eating patterns to look for when you keep a food journal. The first is called *grazing*. Picture a cow grazing . . . all day she is chewing grass. We know, it's not a flattering visual, but that picture is similar to what some overeaters do! They eat all day, with a little here and a little more there—never really eating huge amounts at once, but continuously eating, all day long. Physical hunger is not what motivates grazing. This type of eating happens because food is available or it sounds good at the time.

A second pattern is to overeat during any particular eating episode. According to Jane's journal, she ate two helpings of lasagna instead of one. At the end of the second helping, she felt uncomfortable, but she continued to eat. *Overeating* is when you eat past a feeling of being full or to the point of feeling uncomfortable. A third pattern is *binge eating*, which involves uncontrolled eating episodes in which a person consumes a large number of calories in a short amount of time. Usually bingeing is secretive and occurs when the person is alone; often this type of eating ends with feelings of disgust and a very uncomfortable physical feeling. Bingeing obviously results in weight gain and, in many cases, weight fluctuations. Emotionally, this type of eating leads to feelings of depression, anxiety, low self-esteem, powerlessness, anger, fear, numbness. Social withdrawal and isolation, as well as a social preoccupation with food, are also common. The secrecy involved produces additional guilt and shame.

Use your food journal as an objective information source for the purpose of helping you identify your overeating habits. At this point in the weight-loss journey, it's best not to judge your eating by subjective feelings—you simply can't trust them to be accurate. And remember, people who consistently record food intake lose weight!

Weight Loss Does Not Equal Happiness

One of the greatest myths people hold is that losing weight will make them happy. Granted, it is true that shedding extra pounds does make a person feel better on the outside. However, losing weight uncovers more than we sometimes imagine. And it isn't always happiness, as Cathy describes in her journal:

This week has been a rough one. Lately I've been thinking about the past through rose-colored glasses. Somehow, I remember being happier and more jovial at 350 pounds. I remember being a social butterfly—loud, crazy, and extremely talkative—always looking for spontaneous fun! Sort of like a female John Candy. Boy, have I changed! Without the white stuff (sugar), my personality now is nothing like the one I describe.

Bottom line: I have somehow manipulated my memories into believing that being fat was fun, and I know this isn't true. I guess I'm looking for a good reason to sabotage my new healthy lifestyle. I need help on this one!

What Cathy is experiencing happens to most people who lose as much weight as she has—other issues begin to surface. Cathy is making significant changes and finding out why permanent weight loss is so difficult. Keeping the weight off requires changes in thinking and doing. Once she stopped using food to numb her feelings, past memories began to creep in, memories she had previously avoided. Happily, she was able to analyze what was happening.

Past hurts are usually the root reasons why a person begins to overeat in the first place. The good news is that the root reasons can be healed. Cathy is at a crossroads. If she chooses to confront the reality of her life, she won't feel happy all the time. But if she will learn to deal with those past hurts (and eventually move on), she will no longer need food as a cover-up and she will maintain a healthy weight.

It's easy to be a social butterfly when you are overweight because being fun and jovial is an acceptable way to cover negative feelings. In the same way, it's often easier to laugh and be the life of the party and avoid the reality of hurts and bruised feelings. If you see yourself doing this, you haven't yet taken the red pill. In Cathy's case, as she peels away the excess weight, she is peeling away her old defenses. What's left is the reality . . . the pain she has feared facing. For some overweight people, the past is full of hurtful experiences that were never resolved.

One woman struggles with her weight because her past includes sexual abuse. As she gains control of her compulsive overeating, sexual abuse memories surface. The feelings are intense; she is angry, hurt, and anxious. All kinds of emotions are flooding her as she faces the reality of a past she didn't want to face. Like Cathy, she is at a crossroads. She must face the emotional pain or go back to old habits. The amazing thing is that if she faces those wounds, they can be healed. The woman she was created to be can and will surface. She is living proof of the grace of God demonstrated in Isaiah 61:2-3:

> GOD sent me to announce the year of his grace—
> a celebration of God's destruction of our enemies—
> and to comfort all who mourn,
> To care for the needs of all who mourn in Zion,
> give them bouquets of roses instead of ashes,
> Messages of joy instead of news of doom,
> a praising heart instead of a languid spirit.

Rename them "Oaks of Righteousness"
planted by GOD to display his glory. (MSG)

Happy All the Time

In my (Steve's) book *Toxic Faith*, I address a faith issue that is actually a fat issue for many. One problem people have with Christianity is that they are offered some false promises if they surrender their lives to Jesus. They are told that everything changes and happiness is the result, but this is simply not true. Becoming a Christian does not mean everything will immediately change. Real-life residue is present that must be processed out of our lives. And there are some realities like loss, struggle, temptation, and betrayal that cause us to be anything but happy.

I (Dr. Linda) remember singing a song in Sunday school when I was very young. The boys would karate chop their way through the action motions and the girls would watch and sigh because those young males weren't doing it right! But the lyrics are a little disturbing when I think about them now. Go ahead and do the motions as you sing with me:

I'm in-right, out-right, up-right, down-right happy all the time.
I'm in-right, out-right, up-right, down-right happy all the time.
Since Jesus Christ came in, and cleansed my heart from sin,
I'm in-right, out-right, up-right, down-right happy all the time.

Now don't misunderstand, I am *thrilled* that Jesus came into my life. But the idea of being happy all the time leads me to believe it's time for the red pill! We are *not* happy all the time. We have to learn to deal with difficulty and affliction. We may have to grieve the losses of a less-than-perfect family, or a disappointing marriage, or children making bad choices, or suffering critical and controlling bosses. The important thing to remember is this: You can learn to tolerate bad feelings, to walk through them and let go of them. Or you can overeat and numb out those feelings while gaining weight. And you may need counseling to walk you through those difficult times. That's OK. Walking through the pain is better than avoiding it.

Many new Christians are so disappointed, so broken by the falsehoods of faith not coming through what they heard about or were promised. They eat to comfort and soothe their loss of heart. Fulfillment, purpose, meaning, and security—this is what we have in our relationship with Christ. We do not and should not expect to have happiness for every moment of the rest of our lives.

Lose the Unrealistic Expectations

Thinking your life will be happy if you lose weight is only one of many unrealistic expectations concerning weight loss. Reevaluating your expectations is both necessary and an important part of accepting reality. Here are seven general expectations to reconsider:

1. ALL I HAVE TO DO IS LOSE WEIGHT. Nothing more will be required. This isn't true in most cases. Usually there are reasons you've gained weight unrelated to hunger. Uncovering the reasons why you overeat and then making changes will be required for most people to be successful on a long-term basis.

2. ALL KINDS OF OPPORTUNITIES WILL COME TO ME WHEN I LOSE WEIGHT. We can't tell you how many times this thought sets up disappointment. We've worked with people who believed that, after losing the weight, their dating lives would explode. They were so disappointed when this didn't happen. Other potential opportunities that might be expected include new job opportunities, healed marriages, and blossoming friendships. It's not that these things can't happen, but they

have less to do with losing weight and more to do with how you act and feel about yourself.

3. I WILL LIKE MYSELF BETTER WHEN I'M THINNER. Reality check! Red pill time! You may like yourself less for a short time as you confront things about you that need changing! As Cathy reminded us, losing weight can mean letting go of a significant way to cope with stress and painful memories. And it can also take away your excuse not to work on you. You can hide behind the weight and blame your life on being "fat," or you can face the not so nice parts of yourself and make changes. For example, your office worker may pass you up for a party invitation because you are insensitive, not because you are overweight. Ouch! But as you make necessary changes, you will really like who emerges!

4. I'LL BE GIVING UP A GOOD THING. Food is a poor substitute for community and connection. In the end, it brings neither and leaves you more disconnected than ever. We long to be a part of something bigger than ourselves, to have people who love and care for us, as well as find the one thing that truly feeds us emotionally and spiritually. We won't find these things in food. They can only be found through connection with God and others.

5. I MUST BE PERFECT FOR GOD TO WORK IN ME. Holding this thought, we tend to cover up problems and be dishonest about our struggles because we think God is looking for perfection in order to work. But the reality is that He invites you to be His with every cellulite wrinkle and flaw. One of the problems of the modern church is that we are often taught to cognitively fix things by declaring a Scripture like John 8:32, "Then you will know the truth, and the truth will set you

free." This scripture is absolutely right on! But we need to read the one before it as well (v. 31), "To the Jews who had believed him, Jesus said, 'If you hold to my teaching, you are really my disciples.'" Jesus is telling us that the truth cannot just be read, but must be lived out in our lives—following His commands, loving one another, seeing ourselves as He says we are, picking up our daily cross and following Him, crucifying the flesh, etc. Do you see the difference?

The living truth says no to self and selfish desires and requires an authentic life lived out with others and before the Lord. The truth transforms us, but we have to cooperate during the process in order to look like the Christ who does the transforming. Sadly, we see little of this transformation in our churches because the church often penalizes us for being honest. Problems are hidden as we are encouraged to hang onto Jesus and put on a happy face (and sing that song!).

Interestingly, God didn't hide truth in His Word. For instance, even though it wasn't pretty, the story of the first biblical family (the one with the original problem with choosing the wrong food to eat) involved murder. Throughout the Bible there are unflattering details of sins committed by biblical characters, and yet God so loved the world that He gave His only begotten Son (John 3:16). This is powerful. God sees our imperfections and is able to transform us anyway! But we have to let Him do His work!

6. I'VE SCREWED UP SO MANY TIMES, IT'S JUST TOO LATE. It's never too late with God. Repeat this twenty times until it sinks into your thick skull! God doesn't hold grudges and He certainly doesn't keep on punishing you for sins already confessed. He forgives and calls you to Him. When you accept guilt and shame from your past, you basically tell God that His sacrifice didn't matter. Jesus Christ has taken all your guilt and shame to the cross and doesn't want you holding onto it. He

says, "I'll take your failures and build your future." And He has a great one planned for you.

Witness the life of Peter. Jesus knew Peter would deny Him and lie about being one of His disciples when the going got tough. And when it did, Peter failed miserably. Yet Peter was the man upon whom Jesus chose to build His church. If that doesn't get you excited, we don't know what will!

And we love the fact that, later, Jesus gives Peter three chances to redeem himself personally to the Lord: "When they had finished eating, Jesus said to Simon Peter, 'Simon son of John, do you truly love me more than these?' 'Yes, Lord,' he said, 'you know that I love you.' Jesus said, 'Feed my lambs.' Again Jesus said, 'Simon son of John, do you truly love me?' He answered, 'Yes, Lord, you know that I love you.' Jesus said, 'Take care of my sheep.' The third time he said to him, 'Simon son of John, do you love me?' Peter was hurt because Jesus asked him the third time, 'Do you love me?' He said, 'Lord, you know all things; you know that I love you'" (John 21:15-17). We have to believe that Jesus asks him three times just to correct those earlier three denials. He wanted Peter restored, not punished. That's our God—using our failures and redeeming our losses. But we've got to be honest and not hide our faults and struggles.

7. I CAN DO THIS ALONE. Perhaps this is the mother of all unrealistic expectations. If you could do it alone, you would have by now. Going it alone feeds your appetite. God uses connections to heal us. Going it alone is just a very long and painful path to going right back to where you were before.

Judged by Others but Not by God

Unfortunately, you are judged by your weight. People will think you lack willpower and self-discipline. Have you ever heard, "Just stop putting the food in your mouth"? And don't you want to scream back, "If it were that easy, I'd be at my ideal weight right now!" So what's the lesson? You won't always find the acceptance you desire from other people. Because they are human, they have the potential to fail you. And you can't control what people think or say. Therefore, it's important to find a few people who do understand the battle you are in and who won't judge you, but will pray and encourage you. We'll talk more about this later. But for now, we want you to begin this journey with people who will encourage, love, and accept you.

If you are having trouble finding those people, join our community at www.loseitforlife.com. This Web site is a wonderful resource for weight loss. And remember, God is always with you. His Word is a great source of encouragement. In prayer, say, "God, I refuse to accept words such as lazy, ugly, or out-of-control (fill in the blank) as definitions of who I am. With Your help, I will discover the true me. You created me and declared Your creation good."

Scriptures which declare who you are in Christ are a wonderful source of comfort and support. Put them on 3 x 5 cards or do whatever you need to do to be reminded of your true worth—whatever gets it in your head. You are not what you weigh. You have worth just because God created you. He esteems you already. He's not waiting for you to lose ten pounds. He values you now! He chose you, and He loves you unconditionally. Nothing you do impresses Him. He looks at your heart, not your outward appearance (see 1 Samuel 16:7).

Losing weight doesn't make you more acceptable to God, but unfortunately it influences the judgment of other people. However, don't make the opinions of others a motivation to lose weight. Anytime you try to lose weight for other people, it's a setup for failure.

We are fans of fantasy, but not when it's used for your body and health. Save it for the movies, a great novel, or some other outlet! A good, hard-hitting look at reality isn't as scary as you might imagine. We are going to walk you through it so you face life with your eyes wide open. You can make good decisions when you become aware of what you are doing and then stay aware. If you are used to answering questions about why you overeat with answers like, "I don't know" or "I just wasn't thinking," prepare to have better answers after reading this book. The choice to overeat will still be yours, but it won't be an unconscious choice!

With each Lose It For Life Institute, I begin the sessions with a reality check for those present. Living between expectations and reality brings misery. We must alter our expectations to coincide with reality, a step that will remove misery from our lives. Understand, we can't live every moment without pain, as difficulties do happen, but we can live without misery. Personal desires to be healed by a quick fix or instant solution, or by working harder or just praying more, only give us more misery and more excuses when we fail yet again and reach for food to comfort us. Instead, we need to walk in reality.

Walk in the reality of your needs and expect God to act on your behalf. His way may not always be what you expect, but He can be trusted to intervene. The assurance we have that nothing could ever separate us from God's love is based on His past and present actions on our behalf. Christ sits and pleads our case to the Father; He is always interceding for us on our behalf. "What then shall we say to these things [the reality of our life]? If God is for us, who can be against us?" (Romans 8:31 NKJV).

There are no shortcuts. Body weight is controlled by the number of calories you eat and the number of calories you use each day; that is the reality of taking the red pill. To lose weight, you need to take in fewer calories than you consume. The bottom line is that simple. This happens by becoming more physically active and eating less. Lose It For Life will help you lose the weight and keep it off by sharing suggestions for change in your physical activity and eating habits that will stay with you the rest of your life. Along the way may come changes to your lifestyle, a new awareness of your body, and counsel to deal with potential issues that might keep you from losing the weight permanently.

If you're ready, the time is now. Will you take the red pill? If so, welcome to a new Matrix—Lose It For Life!

3
— Lose Dieting (for Life!) —

Help! I could write a book on dieting. I don't know if there is one I haven't tried. I could fill a garage sale with all the books I've purchased. Maybe I should stack them up and use them for shelves or plant stands and find some real use for them. All kidding aside, I'm tired, broke, and still overweight. For some reason, I keep trying to lose weight. Do you think I've just missed the diet that will really work for me? Which diet do you recommend?

—DESPERATE RITA

Desperate Rita,
There is only one word to answer your question: NONE!

We can't think of anything more depressing than dieting. Who wants to willingly embark on a life of deprivation and eating food you don't enjoy? Just mentioning the word is depressing. We can almost hear your groans and moans, "Not another diet!" Any word that contains this three-letter word—DIE—can't be good.

Dieting Means Deprivation
See if this self-dialogue doesn't ring some familiar bells:

"OK, it's 7:00 a.m. and I'm going to be really good today. I won't eat one piece of candy or one french fry. I will be perfect starting today and get that thin body that will change my life."

By 8:30 a.m. you are hungry and eat two hardboiled eggs (leftovers from Easter on Sunday) out of the refrigerator. Right after you've consumed them, you say: "What is wrong with me!? I already blew my diet. I shouldn't have eaten those eggs! I can't believe I did this. Eggs were not on my list of acceptable foods. I can't even control myself for one day . . . I don't care anymore." Enter [stage left] shame and despair.

By 9:00 a.m. you stare at the candy in the Easter basket and say, "I might as well eat it, too, since I already blew it." You overeat and actually binge on the candy, thereafter becoming disgusted again. "I need a diet that will make me stop eating so much! OK, here is my plan. I'm going to eat grapefruit every day for two weeks. I'm ready. I'm psyched."

Weight loss (mostly water) begins quickly but then slows down after several days. You now add paper-thin crackers and low-fat bars to the grapefruit diet. Both taste like cardboard. And all you can think about is what you can't eat because what you are eating isn't satisfying at all. Then, you remember. There is Ben and Jerry's Cookie Dough™ Ice Cream in the freezer. *It definitely doesn't taste like cardboard.* You dive into the pint and quickly inhale all of it. The eating binge has begun.

"I am really bad. I have no willpower or self-control. Who am I kidding? I really need to get a serious diet. I can't make food choices. Maybe I should try liquids for a week. There has to be something more drastic out there to help me. I've got to get this weight off fast."

A liquids-only diet for one week really does the trick. You lose ten pounds. The weight is dropped! You go off the liquids. Gradually, over a few weeks, all the weight is regained, with five extra pounds being added to the ten that were lost and then gained. It's a vicious cycle. Your life feels out of control, hopeless, and depressing.

Dieting sets up most people to fail. It is not the solution to losing weight and keeping it off. The cycle of depriving yourself, then giving in, then feeling guilty, which leads to more overeating, is classic. The feelings of failure and shame are inevitable. Beating yourself up for not being able to fix the problem leads to a negative self-obsession mode. You are powerless to do what needs to be done—to address the reasons *why* you overeat in the first place.

We should make dieting a disorder and call it what it is—Dieting Disorder (DD)! Don't keep doing this to yourself. Food is not your enemy. Diets, however, make food your enemy. And the dieticians' mantra continues to sound: "There are no forbidden foods." Anything in moderation will not make you fat! Sensible choices combine with practicing moderation in all things while eating foods that have good nutritional content. It should be added that balance and moderation are keys not only to healthy eating, but keys to good living. Both are biblical principles.

> Moderation is better than muscle, self-control better than political power. (Proverbs 16:32 MSG)

> Let your moderation be known unto all men. The Lord is at hand. (Philippians 4:5 KJV)

We must think differently when it comes to choosing food that makes us feel good and is good for us. We need to consider the whole picture. Here's an example from Dr. Linda's life. My children just had their week of SAT testing in school. I made sure they had some protein each morning to feed their brains—they needed foods that would stay with them for a few hours while they concentrated. Though they would have eaten sugary cereal given that option, they needed nutritious food that would sustain them and help them test well. I reminded them there was no good nutrition in sugary cereal and that they would be asleep at their desks in two hours if they made that choice. They agreed and wisely decided to eat a balanced breakfast—proving that even kids can be sensible when it comes to choosing healthy foods.

Dieting Doesn't Fill the Empty Place

Another problem with dieting is that it usually doesn't accomplish what we really need it to do. One of the biggest disappointments is that overeating doesn't fill the emotional needs we have. Yet, how many of us overeat because we have emotional needs or want something? As much as we try, food doesn't fill those empty spaces.

When I (Steve) lost weight in my college days (the most at one time), I did it on a low-carb plan. The weight came off quickly, but it also went back on quickly. It was more of a roller coaster than a yo-yo as there were many twists and turns. But the weight always came back because of two disconnection factors: disconnection from God and disconnection from others. I was an independent loner and rather than work through this chronic problem, I prided myself on my identity. The emptiness of my life drove me back to food over and over again.

So, yes, the low-carb diet worked to get the weight off, but *it didn't keep it off*. It failed to deliver me from a life of obesity and poor health. That state of being only came when I put into place the other factors that would fill the emptiness and heal the emotional conflicts I was experiencing.

To keep the weight off, eventually you have to fill the emptiness with something other than food and start to resolve the emotions. Here's an example: You overeat because you were rejected for a job. As you stuff down the food, your emotions slide right down with it. At the end of this small binge, the rejection is still with you. All that's been accomplished is you have overeaten and numbed out the problem temporarily with food. What really needed to be done was to deal with the rejection. Not getting the job was a loss that must be contended with; it hurt not to be picked.

Perhaps there were things you did in the interview that ruined your chances. Or the interviewer discriminated against you because you were overweight. Or you were under- or overqualified and weren't a viable option. Or perhaps this was not the job for you and God has something better waiting! Whatever the reason, overeating doesn't make the problem go away. At the end of the day, you are still jobless and have overeaten. Overeating actually may compound your bad feelings and make the situation even more painful as feelings of guilt, shame, and failure follow.

Sometimes overeating is triggered because we feel empty. We can feel empty because of unmet emotional needs. Another reason is because we have no active, living relationship with God. We don't go to God with our hurts as He instructs us to do. We don't call on Him for help when we feel helpless. Or we don't trust Him to help us handle our difficult feelings, and so we indulge in an activity that covers the pain. We eat to fill the void, cover the void, or pretend it isn't really there.

Our culture rarely suggests God as an answer to combating feelings of emptiness. Instead, it promotes materialism and false solutions. It tells us we need more—more food, more sex, more cars, bigger homes—more and more stuff, and super-sized! The message is shouted, advertised, sold, and publicized again and again: *More stuff is the answer to your longings.* Empty? Get more!

The truth is that only a personal, intimate relationship with God can satisfy the emptiness we feel. We were created to want more of God. Apart from God, we won't find satisfaction. And He doesn't leave us without a way to satisfy that longing. In addition, the emptiness must be filled with caring people who can love and support us through difficulty. Filling up with things is a poor substitute for relationships and intimacy. Through community and relationships we meet our needs for love and intimacy. This is a point we will make throughout LIFL because it is so important. You cannot be alone and isolated as you take this road to losing it for life.

Dieting Means Missing Something

Diets promote us to miss something based on the premise that we may never be able to eat it again. Sound familiar? Let's say it's Christmas and you pass the buffet table at the office Christmas party. It's loaded with your favorite chocolate éclairs. Usually the thinking goes like this: *It's Christmas. I only get these once a year. I'll need to eat one, no . . . two, or three! After all, it'll be an entire year before I see these again. I can't let this chance pass.* Two weeks later you are at a baby shower. The cake has your favorite frosting, rich cream cheese. *Oh, can you believe this? I'm on a diet and I can't eat that cake. It's right in front of me and I can't have it. Everyone will enjoy the taste but me. I will miss out . . . I better grab it while I can.* One month later, you are in Chicago for business. You pass by Giordano's™ Pizza, home of the best stuffed pizza you've ever tasted. *I can't be in Chicago and not eat Giordano's™ pizza. That would be a crime! But I'm dieting. Even though I could order a small single pizza, I would miss eating all I wanted this one time. I'll get the big stuffed pizza and take the rest back to my hotel for later.* Of course, none of the pizza makes it back to the hotel!

Lose this mentality and lose it for life! When you diet, you keep restricting yourself in ways that set you up to fail. Dieting means you'll be missing the good stuff, when in fact you could have just a taste, or just one piece, or just one slice of the good stuff. You wouldn't gain ten pounds. But thinking you are going to miss out on something sets you up to overeat. What you can't have, you want. This idea goes all the way back to the Garden of Eden. Adam and Eve were given the freedom to eat from any tree in Paradise, except the Tree of the Knowledge of Good and Evil. That was the one tree Adam was told to avoid. When the serpent came to tempt Eve, he began by questioning what God had instructed. He sowed doubt in Eve's mind. The very tree Adam and Eve were to avoid, they ultimately ate from! Think about it. They could have eaten from any tree but one! Eve was deceived and thought she was missing out on something, and Adam disobeyed with her. From the beginning, dealing with restriction has been a problem.

There is always a choice: to eat a food, eat less of it, or skip eating it entirely. A little of something may satisfy our want. The problem is we eat without thinking and focus on what we might be missing. Again, like sin, a little of something forbidden usually ends up being highly desirable. Rather than being self-governed, we give in to the temptation.

Please remember there are no "bad foods" (well, perhaps there are no bad foods other than the deep fried Twinkies™ at your local fair), but there are wise choices. Actually this is a grown-up idea. Most people over twenty-one can have anything they want, but this doesn't mean they should indulge in everything just because they can. There are activities we should choose to do in moderate amounts, like watching TV or sports, and others we should do more often, like playing with our children. Finally, there are other things we shouldn't do at all, like viewing pornography. In every case, we have a choice. Though we don't have to miss a thing if we don't want to, it is very important to note that though everything may be available to us, it is definitely not all good for us. This is especially true of food.

Let's study this example: A mother complained that she couldn't give up eating ice cream. The reason was that her family stopped regularly at an ice cream parlor after each of her children's soccer games. She would sit at the table, drinking her diet drink and pretending she was having fun. But the more she thought about the taste and what she was missing, the more she wanted ice cream. After the kids were delivered home, she returned to the ice cream parlor, alone, and ordered a big hot fudge sundae. She ate it quickly so no one would see her. Feeling slightly sick to her stomach afterward, she rode home and lied about her absence. Then guilt set in as she felt terrible for lying and being so secretive.

Her mistake in choosing not to eat any ice cream is the reason she ended up at the ice cream parlor by herself. It would have been better for her to order a moderate treat with her family present, or divide a sundae with another person, or take a few bites from her husband's ice cream and not feel like she was left out of the fun and celebration. Using moderation, she could have participated. Life isn't usually about all-or-nothing choices. There is a lot of gray area in between. In this case, her choices weren't limited to eating an entire super-sized hot fudge sundae (black) or drinking a diet drink (white). The "gray" included options to divide a sundae, take a few bites, order a small sundae, or to cut back on a dessert later. Or she could say to herself, *I could have a hot fudge sundae, but I choose not to. Later I'll be upset adding those extra calories. It's not worth it to me now.* Thus her decision to not have ice cream would not be made based on feelings of deprivation but feelings of certainty that she would regret her choice.

I (Steve) get kidded often about my ice cream and frozen yogurt strategy. People have told me they just could not do it, but they could if they practiced. The strategy is to always order a child's cone. I will even say to the person making a cone, "Not too much." Then, once I have paid for the treat, I ask anyone if they would like any of it. If the answer is yes, I spoon off the top and give it to them. If I have no takers, I walk over to the nearest trash can and spoon half of it into the trash.

That might seem wasteful to you, but it isn't. I own the cone. It is mine and I am free to do whatever I want with it. If I eat more than I need or want, it does not help one hungry person in Ethiopia. My throwing away a portion of it rather than eating it does not hurt people who are starving either. Each time I do this, I make an adult decision that I do not need the whole cone to feel satisfied. But I know that if I start eating right away (before getting rid of half the ice cream), it will be difficult to stop at the halfway point, or at any point. So I lessen the damage right up front, enjoy the half that I eat, and don't feel deprived at all. In fact, I walk away having had something I really enjoyed while also being proud that I implemented a strategy that worked. It may seem strange, but it's a pretty easy way to save yourself a lot of calories and carbs over a year's time while still enjoying ice cream now and again.

Dieting Gives the Control to Others Instead of You

Another problem with dieting is that you constantly give the control of your food over to others. The diet is like big brother watching your every move. Imagine him saying, "Ah, Sally, you can't have that! No, those chips are not on my plan. Stop eating that pasta—do you see it written on our plan?" Sally, feeling deprived and frustrated by the diet, tells the voice to be quiet and to stop telling her what to do!

Add this internal voice to the myriad expert voices telling you to eat only low fat . . . *no,* high protein . . . *no,* low carbs . . . *no,* high carbs . . . *no,* only vegetables . . . *no!* It's enough to make any of us throw in the towel and say, "Forget it! I'll do what I want to do!"

Chapter six will help you learn to eat what's right for you, to pay attention to your body and how you feel when you eat certain foods, and to make your own choices. Eating is something you do for life. Thus, you need to be in charge of it and not dependent on what others tell you to do. This doesn't mean you can't learn more about nutrition and healthy eating, as it's important to be well informed. But you must learn to make your own decisions and not be so dependent. If you need to enlist the help of a dietitian or nutritionist for awhile, that's fine. He or she can instruct you as to how to eat healthy and sensible meals. Or you can follow our guidelines. But ultimately, you need to feel in control of your choices and be a grown-up who makes your own choices.

Dieting Sets You Up for Bingeing

A serious concern with dieting is that it sets you up to binge, which involves uncontrolled eating episodes in which you consume a large number of calories in a short amount of time, and usually in secrecy.

You may relate to Jim's story. Jim was a rather successful salesman who spent a great deal of time on the road traveling for his job. He decided to diet after gaining a substantial amount of weight. He was motivated by his desperation to meet someone and settle down.

Because Jim traveled so much, most evenings were spent in a hotel room preparing his sales pitches for the next day. The evenings were boring and Jim was anxious. He knew the dangers of pornography and avoided porn movies and videos he could view in his room. His father was an alcoholic, so Jim stayed clear of the hotel bars. But when he was bored and needed a break from the monotony and loneliness of his weeknights, he'd make runs to local grocery stores. There he'd load up on goodies—mostly sweets and desserts.

Night after night, he binged and watched his weight steadily climb. For Jim, bingeing became habitual and was always accompanied by self-loathing. No woman would want him, he reckoned. He was obese and out of control. The key issue, however, was that Jim struggled with loneliness and didn't know how to deal with it. Dieting was his solution. The binges followed. He felt powerless over the food, but the truth is that his powerlessness was directly related to his perceived inability to find a wife and have the life he desired.

A Proper View of Eating

Since there is so much distortion in our culture concerning food, it's best to look at God's original intention for eating. Obviously, He created us with a physical need to eat and provided food as a way to satisfy that need. So what does the Bible say about diets, eating, drinking, overeating, and indulgence in general?

Eating and drinking were common points of fellowship in biblical days. People held feasts, celebrated weddings, invited guests for meals, and used food to nourish, strengthen, and celebrate. The Gospels record Jesus eating meals with His disciples (including the Last Supper), sharing a meal with Lazarus, and being fed by Martha. There is nothing sinful about eating. In fact, eating is often associated with celebration.

Food and drink were used for miracles—Jesus turned water into wine at a wedding and fed thousands of hungry people with loaves and fishes. In Mark, Jesus likened the coming of His kingdom to a wedding feast. In the Old Testament, several feasts are recorded to commemorate Israel's deliverance from Egypt as well as from the wilderness. These occasions symbolized consecration and devotion to God. The first fruits of harvest were dedicated to make atonement for sins and to rejoice and give thanks with the completion of another harvest.

All throughout the Bible, food is discussed symbolically as well as literally and is enjoyed and celebrated. However, like most things, eating and drinking can be excessive. When appetite is ravenous and unrestrained, the Bible calls it *gluttony.* A glutton, according to Webster's dictionary, is described as someone who eats excessively and is greedy or excessively indulgent. So what can we learn from Scripture about gluttony, a topic that is rarely discussed in the modern American church?

Let's face the reality: How many sermons have you heard on this topic? I have counted three in my lifetime. All three were from one series on the Seven Deadly Sins (preached in a Protestant church). Most of you know that the list (as it is) originated in the Catholic Church with Pope St. Gregory the Great. The sins are called "deadly" because they wound love and are considered harmful to one's relationship with God and others. Gluttony is often contrasted with the spiritual virtues of faith and temperance.

The point of understanding gluttony in this context is that it can impede one's spiritual progress or hinder a victorious spiritual life. The Seven Deadly Sins are not a formal list in the Bible, but each one is referenced within the Bible between the books of Genesis and Revelation.

Gluttony Brings Poverty

One of the direct references to gluttony is found in Proverbs 23, a chapter about the importance of exercising restraint. In Proverbs 23:2-3, Solomon instructs, "Don't gobble your food, don't talk with your mouth full. And don't stuff yourself; bridle your appetite" (MSG). In verse 21 of that same chapter, he goes on to say, "Drunks and gluttons will end up on skid row, in a stupor and dressed in rags." In other words, when you don't exercise restraint over eating, the outcome is negative! The message here is don't overindulge. It's true—too much of a good thing is too much!

Gluttony Is a Negative Behavioral Characteristic

Note the reference to gluttony in Matthew 11:19 (MSG). Jesus is talking about how the people tried to discredit Him as Messiah by calling Him a glutton: "I came feasting and they called me a lush, a friend of the riff-raff. Opinion polls don't count for much, do they? The proof of the pudding is in the eating." In this case, gluttony was referred to as a negative behavioral trait. Though feasting was not a problem, becoming a lush was. The intent was to criticize Jesus by calling Him a glutton, someone who couldn't bridle His appetite or exercise control over His life. It's ironic that the Pharisees applied this label to Christ, who is God. He is in total control. There is nothing "excessive" about Him! Those Pharisees didn't like that and so resorted to name-calling, a rather childish maneuver.

Gluttony Is Rebellion

A warning against rebellion is found in Deuteronomy 21:18-21, which speaks to the fallout of a rebellious son in a family. "When a man has a stubborn son, a real rebel who won't do a thing his mother and father tell him, and even though they discipline him he still won't obey, his father and mother shall forcibly bring him before the leaders at the city gate and say to the city fathers, 'This son of ours is a stubborn rebel; he won't listen to a thing we say. He's a glutton and a drunk'" (MSG). Amazingly, the punishment for this was to be stoned to death! Go ahead and thank God for His grace and mercy right now! There are no recorded instances of parents having done this in the Old Testament. The consequence was meant to deter rebellion. Apparently it worked well. It surely would have made us obedient!

The point of this biblical chapter isn't to provide an extreme model for solving rebellion today. We live under the New Covenant in which mercy and grace are freely extended. (Breathe a sigh of relief with us!) We believe, however, that this chapter underscores an important truth —rebellion to family, to proper authority, and to God ultimately leads to destruction and negative consequences—consequences God wanted the children of Israel to avoid for their own good. This is wisdom from which to benefit.

Have you ever thought about your eating as rebellion? In some cases, this is a motive for excessive eating. Do you eat when you want to rebel? Are you compliant on the outside but secretly rebelling on the inside? These are important questions to ask yourself, as it is possible to be eating out of a feeling of rebellion. For example, a man who needed to confront his wife for a hurtful remark she made reported eating to "show her." "She wasn't about to control me by what she said," he angrily cried out. When we got down to the motive for his overeating, which was to rebel against what he thought his wife wanted him to be, we made progress. In his heart, he felt rebellious, even though it wasn't apparent from his physical outlook. Later he realized that he was angry with God too. In fact, he blamed God for his unhappy life. His response was to rebel against his wife, body, and God, and to harbor anger and resentment.

Our Bodies Are for the Glory of God

As you read through these biblical references to gluttony, it's easy to see why more ministers don't preach on this topic! It seems negative and depressing. Yet God created your body. He chose you as His. His spirit lives in you. Read 1 Corinthians 6:19: "Or didn't you realize that your body is a sacred place, the place of the Holy Spirit? Don't you see that you can't live however you please, squandering what God paid such a high price for? The physical part of you is not some piece of property belonging to the spiritual part of you" (MSG). What Paul is saying is that our bodies are sacred and what we do with them affects all parts of us. Our bodies are the dwelling places of the Most High God. We need to take care of them and allow them to be used for God's glory. If gluttony is the sin that is preventing us from being used for God's glory, we need to admit it and repent from it, however painful that act may be.

Lose It For Life is not about wishing for a more sensitive world so our lives would be better. It is about transformation. And transformation will only occur when we face the reality of what we are involved in. Not all who have a weight problem are gluttons, so if you aren't, don't feel falsely accused. But if you are struggling with gluttony, admitting it to God and another person could be the first step toward freedom. If God has been replaced with the food idol and you gluttonously worship that idol with all the devotion you can muster, accepting the true nature, degree, and description of the problem is the way to begin transforming.

Anyone's obsession with food can take on an idol-worshiplike proportion. When we worry, think, and obsess about what we will eat, or look forward to meals more than our time with God, we are out of balance. Worry is a distracting trait. If we worry about what we eat, how much we'll be able to have, and how often we can get it, we are not following Christ's directive in Matthew 6:25, "If you decide for God, living a life of God-worship, it follows that you don't fuss about what's on the table at mealtimes or whether the clothes in your closet are in fashion. There is far more to your life than the food you put in your stomach, more to your outer appearance than the clothes you hang on your body" (MSG).

A life decided for God has the promise that God will meet your physical needs as well as your emotional and spiritual ones. Accept the promises. God wants you to enjoy eating yet not become a glutton. These words are not meant to be harsh but to help you understand that anything taken to excess can block a vibrant relationship with God. *Moderation is key.*

You are not condemned by God or us for overeating. God wants to bring you to improved health, to remove your obsession with food, to prevent negative consequences related to your overeating, and to help you enjoy meals and fellowship with others. He wants you to experience the enjoyment of food, the pleasure of taste, and the sensation of a full stomach rather than be bound by guilt, physical discomfort, or negative health consequences related to obesity and bingeing.

The Bible also tells us to get out of spiritual poverty by developing self-control, a fruit of the Spirit (Galatians 5:22), and to submit our entire lives to God "as living sacrifices" (Romans 12:1). Allow Him to use you for His glory—it is a primary reason for why you were created!

Distinguishing Between the Hungers

I eat but I'm not really hungry. At least, I don't think I am. I'm not really sure. Sometimes I feel like I could eat everything in the cupboards, like I'm ravenous. So I just do. I never really think about if I'm hungry or not. I think I just really like food, lots of food. And lots of times, I crave things—like cookies. I'll go to the bakery and pretend to be buying a dozen cookies for my kids at school, but really, I plan on eating them all.

What is hunger? What motivates it? Is the need physical, emotional, or spiritual? The three faces of hunger are very different and often confused, as many of us have discovered. The need for deeper emotional and spiritual fulfillment can be viewed instead as physical hunger. And though there may be immediate gratification when we eat, we will not be truly satisfied unless we are eating to fill a physical hunger.

Physical Hunger

Physical hunger is a normal body sensation, a cue that the body needs refueling. Physical hunger goes away when there is food to satisfy it. Hunger is part of God's creative design. To identify physical hunger, you must learn to recognize the physical sensations that accompany it. Usually hunger builds because you haven't eaten in a while. Your body signals its need for food—whether it is a rumbling, growling, or emptiness in the pit of your stomach. You may also experience low energy or even light-headedness. Eating even a small amount of food usually stops these sensations.

We have other needs apart from our physical bodies. There are the needs to be safe, to belong, to be loved, to be esteemed, and to grow. Emotional hunger relates to an unmet emotional need. Even though emotional needs can't be satisfied by food, that doesn't stop us from trying. Yet as most of us know, this doesn't work. Food is used like a drug, with a purpose of distracting, numbing, and helping us avoid the reality of hurt and pain or the emptiness of an unmet need.

The following table will help you to distinguish differences between physical and emotional hunger[9]:

Physical Hunger	Emotional Hunger
Builds gradually	Hits suddenly, "starving"
Stomach starts to rumble and growl	Anxiety; but there is no real "physical" symptom of feeling hungry
Feel full and stop eating	Overeat even if feeling full
Different foods will satisfy	Crave very specific food; nothing else satisfies
Physically feel empty in pit of stomach	Mouth and mind are tasting the food
Need to eat but can wait	Eat now to ease whatever is happening
Eat and feel fine	Eat and feel guilt and shame
4-5 hours since last meal; feel light headed, low energy	Upset and want to eat now
Choose foods purposefully	Automatic or absentminded eating

If you had difficulty on your food journal deciding whether or not you were physically hungry each time you ate, this exercise may help. The next time you eat, make a guess as to which type of hunger you are experiencing. List the three columns in the following chart. In the first column, check which hunger you think you are having. In the second column, write down your feelings, physical sensations, emotions, and thoughts right before you wanted to eat. In the third column, write down how you felt after you ate. Read what you listed and decide if you checked the correct type of hunger. A blank copy of this chart is provided in Appendix B. Your chart might resemble this one:

Physical or Emotional Hunger?	Before I ate, I felt: *(Feelings and thoughts)*	After I ate, I felt: *(Feelings and thoughts)*
Emotional	Upset and mad, wanted to eat, stomach tense from anger	Tired, immediately uncomfortable
Physical	Ate four hours ago, light-headed, stomach growling	Satisfied, energized

Each time you eat, something precedes the eating. We call these "triggers" or "cues." A trigger or cue signals that something is about to begin. A physical trigger involves a physical symptom—something like feeling short of energy, light-headedness, a growling stomach, headache, or dizziness.

Emotional Hunger

Emotional triggers involve feelings: feeling upset, bored, hurt, angry, disappointed, lonely, happy, etc. If you notice that all your checks are in the emotional column, then we have work to do. The goal is to eat more often in response to physical cues than emotional ones.

If you aren't sure what you are feeling or thinking, here's an additional exercise. Next time you eat, focus on the *experience* of eating and become very aware of your physical and emotional state. The goal is to stay in the moment of eating and avoid eating without thinking.

Sixty seconds before you eat, sit quietly (with no distractions) and think—what do I feel and what am I thinking about right now? Record this. Then look at what you are about to eat. Notice how it tastes. Do you like what you are eating? Do you like the feel of it in your mouth? How does it feel in your stomach? After you finish, take another sixty seconds and write down how you feel—energized, tired, unsatisfied, content, etc.

This short exercise will put you in touch with the experience of eating. It will slow you down and help you pay attention to all the sensations involved in eating. After emotional eating, you'll often feel tired and sluggish or won't feel satisfied because eating wasn't what you needed to do. In addition, when you choose sugary foods, your blood sugar rises and falls quickly, which makes you feel tired. The goal is to find out why you are eating in the first place and to stop eating when you aren't physically hungry.

Why do we eat when we aren't hungry? Sometimes this behavior happens out of habit—such as when food is treated as a reward or involves a celebration. It also serves as a numbing device or plan of avoidance when we feel unpleasant. Often people eat because they feel impulsive and want to gratify those impulses quickly. Other people eat to indulge in something good because they are feeling deprived by other things in life. Whatever the reason, finding out why you are eating is paramount to losing weight and keeping it off. Once you get a handle on why you eat, you can make changes.

At this point, begin to tune in to your physical, mental, and emotional state. Pay attention to the cues that lead to overeating. Write them down and study them. Stay aware and "in the moment" while eating. Soon you'll know the difference between real hunger and emotional hunger.

Spiritual Hunger

During the Sermon on the Mount, Jesus said, "Blessed are you who hunger now, for you will be satisfied" (Luke 6:21). The Greek word for "hunger" is *peinas*, meaning "to be hungry, to be famished, to be starved." Jesus tells us to hunger after Him and we will be satisfied. What we think is hunger for food or even emotional hunger may be a hunger for more of God. We were created with a space for God to live in us, not to be empty. His desire is for us to have life and have it more abundantly. Yet how many of us are satisfied with the scraps from the table when He promises us a feast? We are spiritually starving and don't feed our hunger the right way. We become distracted with other things that won't fill that spiritual void.

Beth Moore says, "Victory is not determined as much by what we've been delivered *from* as by what we've been delivered *to*." She is so right. You won't be victorious over food and overeating unless you look to God to satisfy you. Nothing else will really do. God wants to deliver you from the need to overeat. He wants you to find your purpose, move in His power, and live a life of overcoming. He offers Himself to you. He is your deliverer. With God there is relationship, intimacy, and abundant life, not to mention peace, joy, and so much more! He offers that which will satisfy. Heed His promise! He wants you, chose you, and is waiting to fill your mouth with good things.

When you feel depressed by a gnawing emptiness in your soul, focus on your hope in Christ. God's promises are many, and they are meant to be read and treasured and cried over and praised over. Let these Scriptures encourage you and fill that empty space within you:

> For everything that was written in the past was written to teach us, so that through endurance and the encouragement of the Scriptures we might have hope. —ROMANS 15:4

> May the God of hope fill you with all joy and peace as you trust in him, so that you may overflow with hope by the power of the Holy Spirit.
>
> —ROMANS 15:13

> I pray also that the eyes of your heart may be enlightened in order that you may know the hope to which he has called you, the riches of his glorious inheritance in the saints.
>
> —EPHESIANS 1:18

God has so much more for you. He doesn't want you dragging through life being defeated by your weight. He wants to give you good things—more of His power, more of His Spirit, more of His love and compassion. The urgency you feel to fill up with food, to overeat, could be the Holy Spirit urging you to satisfy your spiritual hunger through God. Are you afraid you won't get what you need? Not to worry. God has enough to go around for all of us. His resources are limitless. He is the Living Water that never runs dry. He is the Bread of Life who promises eternal life. The fullness He has for you cannot be found in the temporal things of this world. And once you experience His fullness, you'll never hunger in the same way again!

So why don't we hunger and thirst after righteousness? Too often it is because we listen to the voice of the accuser. The Bible tells us the accuser is the devil and that he accuses us day and night (Revelation 12:10). Think about it. Satan can't undo our salvation, so he has to have other tricks to trip us up. One of his best schemes is to accuse us with claims that we aren't worthy, we can't lose weight, or that we are all losers. His accusations are constantly ringing in our ears. But we cannot listen to him or believe his lies because we have been cleared of all accusations, as Hebrews 10:19-23 tells us:

So, friends, we can now—without hesitation—walk right up to God, into "the Holy Place." Jesus has cleared the way by the blood of his sacrifice, acting as our priest before God. The "curtain" into God's presence is his body. So let's do it—full of belief, confident that we're presentable inside and out. Let's keep a firm grip on the promises that keep us going. He always keeps his word. (MSG)

Did you grasp that truth? You are cleansed by the blood of Christ's sacrifice. Once you confess sin, there is nothing Satan can do about it because it's no longer there. So he can accuse all he wants. You just tell him to go take a hike because there is nothing left for Satan to accuse. You have to believe this truth and stop letting the devil take your past and hold it up like an autobiography. Yes, you have sinned, but once confessed, the book's pages are blank. There is no record of those wrongs anymore, because the sin has been cleared.

You've got to get this into your spirit and not allow the enemy to steal your joy. Hunger for more of God. God holds all satisfaction. Perhaps you've tried to find satisfaction in many other ways. Rest in the assurance that nothing completely satisfies except more of God. God wants to fill your hungry, empty life with the bread that truly satisfies, and He will—when you sit down for the meal and open your heart and life to His will and His voice.

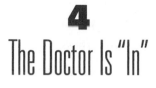

4
The Doctor Is "In"

Early on, we mentioned that one size does not fit all when it comes to losing weight and keeping it off. In this chapter, we want to focus on physical influences that affect weight loss and maintenance. Your physical body is unique and it must be factored in to any program tailored specifically for you. For example, if you have a family history of obesity, you have a greater chance of being obese than someone who does not. This reality doesn't doom you to be overweight, but it is an influence you should recognize.

Whatever your history or genetic picture, be aware that physical influences can speed up or slow down the work. The better informed you are, the more patient you will be with yourself when it comes to achieving your goals. Although you may not be able to control all the factors that led to becoming overweight, you do have control over how you respond to them.

As you consider this chapter, try not to get hung up on the fairness of the genetic hand you may have been dealt. Think of life like a card game—it's not so much the hand you are dealt that influences a win, it's how you play that hand! Your genetic history is part of who you are. Your biology may create more challenges. However, it won't stop you from being successful. By taking care of your body, monitoring your health, and making lifestyle changes, you can and will lose it for life.

Wearing the Genes That Fit

Heredity plays a role in what you weigh. If you have a family history of obesity, pay special attention to your food intake and other factors that affect weight gain, because your chances of becoming obese increase by about 30 percent.[10] Being overweight and/or obese runs in families. Researchers are still trying to decide how much of family obesity is due to shared genes or shared family eating and exercise habits. However, twin studies indicate that genetic factors do play a role. Having overweight family members isn't a guarantee that you'll be overweight, but this fact does increase your chances.

Basal Metabolic Rate

People also inherit basal metabolic rates. Basal metabolic rate (BMR) is the number of calories you would burn if you stayed in bed all day (not a recommendation we are making). The lower the rate, the more difficult it is to lose weight. BMR is affected by height—lower for short versus tall people—and by weight—the more fatty body tissue you have, the lower the BMR. In contrast, the more lean body tissue you have, the higher the BMR. As you will read in chapter seven on exercise, building lean body tissue is one of the goals of regular exercise and can help raise BMR.[11]

As you age, you may begin to gain weight even though your eating habits do not change. This is because the body's metabolism slows down with aging. In other words, your body requires fewer calories to do the same work. So eating the same amount of food without changing your activity level can lead to gradual weight gain.

In addition, fever, stress, heat, and cold all raise BMR. Fasting, starving, and malnutrition lower it. Dieting and skipping meals can trick your body into thinking it is starving—thereby slowing down weight loss instead of increasing it! This is the best reason not to "diet." BMR is regulated by the thyroid hormone thyroxin. The more thyroxin produced, the higher the BMR. This helps explain why a low thyroid slows down weight loss in some people. If you suspect this might be your problem, have it checked.[12] And if you want to find out once and for all if you have a low metabolic rate, you can have it measured by indirect calorimetry. This service is inexpensive and can easily be done at most hospitals (pulmonary department) or by sports medicine clinics. However, low metabolism is usually not the culprit when it comes to weight gain. We know because we have both tried to use it as an excuse for overeating.

When I (Dr. Linda) was a college cheerleader, I was extremely active. There were daily practices and gymnastic classes in addition to games. After road games, the team and cheerleaders would stop at fast food places and load up on food. My fellow cheerleaders ordered shakes, double burgers, and fries. Since they were thin and we had all just exercised vigorously, I figured I could load up on food too and stay thin. Well, I couldn't and began to gain weight. I was sure my metabolism was slower than everyone else's was (even though I never had a problem with it before and was skinny as a child). In reality I needed to take the red pill as I was eating a whole lot more food than the splurges on away-game nights. My metabolism had little to do with my weight gain and more to do with regular late-night eating in the dorm. But for years, I believed I suffered from a low BMR.

I (Steve) had a low BMR growing up that caused me to greatly resent my older brothers, who could eat more than me and remain fit and trim. It didn't seem fair that my body worked against me. But I discovered something that could be a great source of hope for you. My metabolism works for me now. The difference? Then I had little muscle on my frame. Today, after years of regular workouts with weights, I have much more. What I did can work for you! As we age, we lose muscle tissue each year, which lowers our metabolisms. But with weight training and resistance exercises, that rate of loss can be reduced. You can even build muscle tissue and increase your metabolism, enabling you to lose weight easier or to eat more and still maintain the right weight.

Exercise is a gift from God, and it can be utilized to change your future and have one where you are not defined by your weight. There are many things in this world that cannot be influenced or changed on your own power. But you *can* choose to build muscle and raise your own metabolism, which is reason to hope. You can make your body's metabolism work for you rather than against you.

Fat Cell Number and Size

Another physical factor is fat cell number and size. Fat cells begin to triple from birth to six years of age in both boys and girls. The result is a gradual and similar increase in body fat. But after about eight years of age, girls take off at a faster rate than boys. Fat cell size, not number, increases. Between the ages of six and adolescence, fat cell numbers stay constant in normal-weight children. However, in obese children, the number of fat cells can increase. When adolescence hits, girls almost double the rate of increasing fat of boys. More and larger fat cells are increased about the pelvis, buttocks, thighs, and breasts—a phenomena related to female hormonal changes.

In women of healthy weights, fat accumulation more or less stops after adolescence with no further increase in the number of fat cells. Similarly, in post-adolescent males of a healthy weight, fat cells tend not to multiply. You have probably noticed that men tend to store excess fat in their bellies or abdomens. This is a dangerous place to accumulate fat because it is associated with an increased risk in coronary artery disease, elevated triglycerides, hypertension, and cancer.[13] Fat cells that are packed and swell and become large enough to be seen through the skin are called cellulite. As our skin gets thinner with age and becomes less flexible, cellulite becomes more visible. The only help for this is weight loss and regular activity.[14]

Even if a person has a normal number of fat cells, those cells can increase in size and weight throughout life if that person becomes grossly overweight. The number and size of fat cells reflects the amount of fat stored in the body. If you consume more energy than you expend, it is stored in fat cells. When fat cells reach their maximum size, they may divide and create more. Obesity results when fat cells increase in number, size, or both.

If you have a higher than normal number of fat cells in your body, you won't lose fat cells by dieting. Fat cells can shrink, but they don't leave the body. Even if you temporarily manage to empty them, they can easily fill up again as you gain weight. This is why it is easier for someone with an excess of fat cells to gain weight. There is only one way to get rid of fat cells: by liposuctioning them out. And although this may get rid of the fat cells, it's not something we are recommending because it isn't a solution to lifestyle changes that may be needed.

The Stress Factor

You'd have to be living on another planet not to know that stress affects your body in negative ways. One of those negative ways relates to weight gain. While an immediate response to stress may be a loss of appetite, repeated and chronic stress can cause the opposite effect. Here's why.

When you encounter stress, cortisol, along with other hormones, is released. Following a stressful event, the other hormones return to normal levels, but cortisol can remain elevated for a longer time period.

Because this hormone provides energy for the body, it can stimulate appetite and result in weight gain that tends to be concentrated in the midsection or abdominal area.

According to Pamela M. Peeke, M.D., MPH (Masters of Public Health), a former senior scientist at the National Institutes of Health in Bethesda, Maryland, and an associate clinical professor of medicine at the University of Maryland School of Medicine in Baltimore, three factors affect central fat in women. They are poor lifestyle, declining levels of the hormone estrogen, and chronic stress.[15] The amount of cortisol experienced with stress seems to vary from person to person. If you are someone who reacts to stress with increased appetite, you may be experiencing elevated cortisol levels. Whether or not your urge to eat is driven by hormones, you can still interrupt the cycle, break the stress, and stop weight gain. Since stress is something we all experience, we all need to learn effective ways to manage or reduce it. Lifestyle changes recommended in this program can help you with stress.

Begin to evaluate what you are doing that may add stress to your life. Are there habits and practices you could change today that would make you feel better? The answer is probably yes. Think about your response to stress in terms of self-care. How will you take care of yourself in order to battle the negative effects of stress?

1. DO YOU HAVE EFFECTIVE WAYS OF RELAXING? We all need downtime. Relaxation isn't something you do once a year on a cruise to the Bahamas (although this can't hurt). Relaxing should be a regular, practiced part of your life. You need balance in all things. Even God rested on the seventh day! Relaxation keeps stress from building up and provides an avenue for releasing tension.

2. DO YOU REGULARLY EXERCISE? The benefits of exercise are

enormous and an entire chapter will be devoted to the topic as it is an essential ingredient to losing weight for life. Exercise can reduce muscle tension and frustration in addition to providing a host of medical helps. Find something you like—bike riding, dancing, skating, basketball, tennis, skiing, walking, ping pong—anything that gets you off that couch and moving!

3. HOW SENSIBLY DO YOU EAT? Do you eat good food that provides nutrition and health benefits? Do you skip meals? Eat burgers in the car while talking on your cell phone? Find yourself at the drive-thru regularly? Chapter six will address eating habits.

4. HOW WELL DO YOU MANAGE YOUR TIME? So many people spend energy on things that are unproductive or take up too much of their time. If you are not meeting deadlines or procrastinate or obsess over projects, you need help. Some people have to learn to move along more efficiently, while others need to slow down and do things correctly. Because our time is limited, it's important to learn to prioritize and be realistic about goals.

5. ARE YOU GETTING ENOUGH SLEEP? This sounds like a simple question, but so many people have terrible sleep habits. Going to bed at a regular time and getting into a sleep routine is essential. A lack of sleep is associated with changes in hormone levels. When cortisol levels remain high from a lack of sleep, the body craves carbohydrates and foods high in calories and fat. Metabolism then slows down as the body stores fat.[16] And here's an encouraging thought for those to whom it morally applies—sex usually helps people sleep. Now there's a sleep motivator we can live with!

Revisit Your Motivation

We'll say it again: Your motivation for losing weight should not be to please someone else. If you are doing this because your physician or spouse is upset with you, this is a set-up for potential failure. Decide if you are ready to lose weight for your own personal reasons. How important is it to you to live a life undefined by your weight and driven by food and eating? How important is it to you that you lead a healthy life?

*If you are motivated to work on all parts of your life—spiritual, physical, emotional, and interpersonal—you will do well. You must take ownership of your goal to lose weight and keep it off. No one else can do it for you, but with God's help, you can be successful. It is also helpful to ask the question, "Why do I want to lose weight **now**?" Since you have probably dieted in the past and been overweight for months or even years, why are you ready now? Hopefully you are ready to surrender this problem to God and accept the reality of your situation, including taking responsibility for your part of the problem.*

Finally, are you experiencing significant stress right now? If so, this may not be the time to try and lose weight. Instead, you may want to concentrate on making lifestyle changes rather than focusing on weight loss. Significant life stress greatly disrupts a person's ability to lose weight for life. If this resonates with you, please read the material below, and make any lifestyle changes possible, given your current circumstances—any changes that can be made without overtaxing yourself. When your circumstances have stabilized, consider adding a goal of weight loss.

Confronting the Reality of Size and Weight

Another physical factor to consider is how much weight you have to lose. The more you have to lose, the longer it takes. Don't expect to go from 300 pounds to 180 overnight. Begin by setting your weight loss goal at 10 percent of your current body weight, and consider weight loss of one to two pounds a week successful. This is very doable since you can lose weight just by eating 100 calories less a day than you need. Over time, this small reduction will result in a gradual yet steady weight loss.

When you are overweight or obese, the last thing you want to do is confront the reality of your size. To do so means to acknowledge what that state is doing to your physical body. One obese client, an elementary school teacher, experienced great heartache when the reality of her growing size became evident to her. While teaching one day, she suddenly realized that she could no longer fit in the aisles between her students' desks.

When she left school that day, she sat in her car in the parking lot and cried. This experience was a wake-up call. Her overeating was out of control. She knew she was gaining weight but had refused to confront the fact, as many overweight people do. Most look in the mirror from their necks up. They fix their hair, do their makeup, and put on a happy face without looking at the rest of their bodies because it is too painful and depressing. Yet taking a full-length view keeps reality in front of you and can be used as an incentive to make changes.

Rather than look in the mirror and verbally beat yourself up, try this: Stand fully unclothed in front of a full-length mirror. Slowly scan your entire body. Feel the various parts. We know this sounds cruel, but it isn't. The goal is to be in touch with the reality of your size and weight. It's important to your health—another subject that is often avoided by overweight people.

Perhaps you don't want to think about the size of your body or what the extra weight is doing to your overall health, but again, awareness is critical. It is too easy to disconnect your eating from your physical body. Instead, intentionally think about that extra weight and the potential health impact it has, and use this to motivate lifestyle changes, not degrade yourself. To do so is to take a very courageous step, as this journal entry indicates:

Last May I weighed 350 pounds. Today I weigh 237 pounds. Do you have any idea how much easier it is to walk, work, drive, and even sleep with a 113-pound weight loss? Looking back, I am amazed that I was able to function as well as I did. I know laziness is one of the stereotypes for obese individuals, but believe me when I say I have never been a lazy person. I have always been a hard worker, one that ran around the office doing the work of three in hopes of being accepted by the "normal folks."

It was tough weighing 350 pounds. It was hard work carrying the extra pounds everywhere I went. I don't think the world realizes what we go through. The good news for today is that I have given up 113 pounds of baggage (physically and emotionally) and my load is becoming lighter each week. My goal is to have as little baggage as possible. It takes hard work, dedication, and complete faith in Jesus Christ, but He will carry our load if we ask Him.

— CATHY

Cathy had to face the reality of her 350-pound frame. It hurt to even walk. Carrying that weight impacted her ability to do everyday tasks. Furthermore, several doctors told her that she wouldn't live long if she didn't make changes. As a single mom who faced the reality staring back at her, Cathy decided she had to do something about it.

Let's Get a Physical

I can't go for a physical. It's too humiliating. Last time I tried (years ago), the doctor never looked me in the eye. I could tell he was disgusted with me. The exam was quick and he barely touched me. Then he handed me a 1,200-calorie diet and told me to lose weight, stating matter-of-factly that my weight would probably kill me. I was ashamed and embarrassed. I've tried his diet but can't do it. I

*do have heart disease in my family, so he wants me to come back. I
don't want to go again. I'd rather not think about it.*　　—SUE

A comprehensive physical examination conducted by a competent
physician is necessary to obtain an accurate picture of your health. You
do need that physical. However, we advise that you change doctors if
you are uncomfortable with your current physician. Happily, Sue did;
a follow-up physical by a new doctor revealed that she had type 2 diabetes. She needed medical supervision and intervention.

We suggest you find a physician who is compassionate and sensitive
to overweight people. Unfortunately, we've heard too many stories like
Sue's in which physicians simply hand patients 1,200-caloric diets and
tell them to lose weight. Reality check: If this worked, people would be
able to follow this advice and drop weight. In our experiences, this
strategy only compounds feelings of failure in an overweight person.

If your physician is insensitive regarding your weight, change doctors and tell your health care company why you are doing so. As an overweight person, you already have to contend with ridicule and stigma
from the public. You don't need to put up with either from your health
care provider. One of my (Dr. Linda's) physicians has a framed plaque
on his wall that I have received permission to copy here. I love what Dr.
Su wrote:

> Let a doctor be called as a healer, not the health care provider.
> Let the patient be treated as the healed, not the health care con-
> sumer.
> Medicine is not a commercial business but a professional practice
> based strongly on a doctor-patient relationship of compassion,
> understanding, and respect.[17]

Find a doctor like Dr. Su who won't treat you like a consumer, but who will show you compassion and be a part of the healing. A physician can monitor your medical conditions, work with you on improving your health, support your efforts to make changes, be aware of the issues involved in your weight loss maintenance, and encourage a holistic approach.

In addition, keep in mind that some illnesses can lead to obesity or a tendency to gain weight. These include hypothyroidism, Cushing's syndrome, depression, and specific neurological problems that can lead to overeating. Also, certain medications may have side effects that cause weight gain, including steroids and some antidepressants. A doctor can evaluate whether there are underlying medical conditions that may be causing you to gain weight or will make weight loss more difficult. This is information you need to know.

The following section lists the health risks commonly associated with being overweight and obese. This list is not comprehensive. It only touches on main concerns. Of course, there may be other health issues or conditions that require medical supervision and treatment as well. This list is not meant to scare you or make you fearful. Knowing that our tendency is to deny health risks, reading this list is a necessary step as we consider our health. Use this information to motivate and to accept the reality of your health if you make no changes. Keep in mind that even modest weight loss improves your health.

Common Health Risks Associated with Being Overweight and Obese

Type 2 Diabetes

This type of diabetes is also referred to as adult onset or non-insulin dependent diabetes and is the most common in the United States. It is a disease in which blood sugar levels are above normal and can cause early death, heart disease, kidney disease, stroke, and blindness.

If you are overweight, your risk for type 2 diabetes increases. In fact, about 80 percent of people with this disease are overweight.[18] One thought is that extra weight may put stress on the cells that produce insulin (a hormone that carries sugar from the blood to the cells). The extra stress may make the cells less effective and cause problems. Losing weight and exercising can lower your risk for type 2 diabetes and possibly reduce your current medication if you are already diagnosed.

Heart Disease and Stroke

Heart disease and stroke are caused when your heart, circulation, or blood flow do not operate normally. When this happens, you can have a heart attack, congestive heart failure, sudden cardiac death, angina (chest pain), or abnormal heart rhythm. Heart disease is the leading cause of death in the United States, and death from a stroke places third.[19]

Being overweight puts you more at risk for factors related to heart disease and stroke, including high blood pressure, high levels of triglycerides, high "bad" cholesterol (LDL), and low "good" cholesterol (HDL). Also, obesity is related to inflammation in blood vessels and throughout the body, which is also a risk for heart disease.[20]

By losing between 5 and 15 percent of your body weight, you can lower your risk for both health problems. Think about it! When as little as ten pounds of weight loss can make a difference, it's really not much weight to lose.

Cancer

Cancer touches all of us in some way and is the second leading cause of death in this country. Perhaps you have a friend or family member suffering from one form or another, or you have been diagnosed with cancer yourself. This disease occurs when cells in one part of the body grow out of control or abnormally. Cancer can spread to other parts of the body as well.

When you are overweight, your risk of developing certain types of cancers increases, including colon, esophageal, uterine, postmenopausal breast cancer (women), and kidney. Researchers aren't sure why being overweight is a factor in increased risk, but one possibility is that fat cells make hormones that might affect cell growth.[21] The current thinking is that preventing weight gain, eating healthily, and being physically active may lower your risk for cancer.

Sleep Apnea

Sleep apnea occurs when a person stops breathing for short periods during the night. The result is usually daytime sleepiness, difficulty concentrating, and even heart failure. Usually weight loss improves this condition because it decreases the neck size and inflammation.[22] Research tells us this condition is more prevalent for people who are overweight. One reason is that an overweight person may have fat stored in the neck area that can make the airway for breathing smaller. These fat stores can also result in the neck becoming more inflamed, which can put a person at a greater risk for sleep apnea. As a result, breathing can be difficult, loud (snoring), or even stop altogether.

Osteoarthritis

This is a joint disorder in which the tissues that protect joint bones and cartilage gradually wear away. Most commonly affected are the joints of the knees, hips, and lower back. The more weight you carry, the more pressure you put on your joints and cartilage. Additional weight may also increase blood levels of body substances that cause inflammation, which may in turn increase the risk for osteoarthritis.

Again, weight loss can remove some of the stress on your knees, hips, and lower back.[23]

Gallbladder Disease

When you are overweight, your risk for gallbladder disease and gallstones increases. This is partly due to the fact that more cholesterol is being produced, which is an associated risk factor. Being overweight can also make your gallbladder enlarged or unable to work efficiently.[24]

If you've ever had a gallstone (a cluster of solid material—mostly cholesterol—that forms in the gallbladder), you know pain! People who lose a lot of weight very quickly (more than three pounds a week) increase their chances to develop gallstones. Often clients who try very low-calorie diets have an increase in gallbladder disease. The message here is to shoot for modest, consistent weight loss of one half to two pounds a week to prevent an increased risk.

Fatty Liver Disease

Even the name of this illness is unappealing! It results from the buildup of fat cells in the liver that causes injury and inflammation. It can cause severe liver damage, cirrhosis (scar tissue in the liver that blocks blood flow), and liver failure. It sounds serious, and it is. Most people know about this condition because of the link it has to alcohol. But you can get this disease without drinking any alcohol when you are overweight. Overweight people who are "prediabetic" (have higher blood sugar) are more at risk. Weight loss helps to control blood sugar, which hopefully helps to avoid the buildup of fat. Avoiding alcohol helps as well.[25]

Establish Your Goal

A great place to begin is to establish goals. In terms of healthy weight loss, determine how much weight you want to lose. As you decide on a number or weight range, your goal should meet the following criteria:

1. SPECIFIC. "I want to be thin" is an example of a non-specific goal. It is too vague. "I'd like to lose twenty pounds" is specific.

2. ATTAINABLE. Select a goal that you can actually reach. For example, if you've been 300 pounds most of your adult life and your lowest adult weight was 190 pounds, then do not select a goal weight of 125 pounds. Most likely, you won't reach that goal. But to set a goal of weighing 190 pounds is reasonable given that you have once achieved that weight as an adult. You can always reset your goal once you've reached 190 pounds if you feel there is more you can lose.

When deciding on a weight loss goal, it helps to review your weight history. Use your lowest adult weight as a guideline. Another good rule of thumb is to make 10 percent of your current weight your weight loss goal. When you reach that goal, you can reset your goal for another 10 percent. In our experience, attainable goals build success and confidence. And the meeting of short-term goals brings a sense of accomplishment along the way.

3. FORGIVABLE. In other words, don't be rigid. Be flexible in case you aimed too high. Be open to renegotiating your goals as you go. And when you falter, give yourself permission to rethink the goal and begin again. Sometimes a goal is difficult to achieve because all the issues that go into making that goal haven't been considered. For many people, successful weight loss and maintenance requires lasting changes in all areas of life, something we don't always think about when we want to lose weight.

Metropolitan Life Insurance Charts[26]

These charts are not the end-all when it comes to determining a healthy weight. They are, however, a good tool with which to estimate what weight might be in a healthy range for you. (For more information on these tables, see endnote.)

Height & Weight Table For Women

Height Feet Inches	Small Frame	Medium Frame	Large Frame
4' 10"	102-111	109-121	118-131
4' 11"	103-113	111-123	120-134
5' 0"	104-115	113-126	122-137
5' 1"	106-118	115-129	125-140
5' 2"	108-121	118-132	128-143
5' 3"	111-124	121-135	131-147
5' 4"	114-127	124-138	134-151
5' 5"	117-130	127-141	137-155
5' 6"	120-133	130-144	140-159
5' 7"	123-136	133-147	143-163
5' 8"	126-139	136-150	146-167
5' 9"	129-142	139-153	149-170
5' 10"	132-145	142-156	152-173
5' 11"	135-148	145-159	155-176
6' 0"	138-151	148-162	158-179

Weights at ages 25-59 based on lowest mortality. Weight in pounds according to frame (in indoor clothing weighing 3 lbs.; shoes with 1" heels).

Height & Weight Table For Men

Height Feet Inches	Small Frame	Medium Frame	Large Frame
5′ 2″	128-134	131-141	138-150
5′ 3″	130-136	133-143	140-153
5′ 4″	132-138	135-145	142-156
5′ 5″	134-140	137-148	144-160
5′ 6″	136-142	139-151	146-164
5′ 7″	138-145	142-154	149-168
5′ 8″	140-148	145-157	152-172
5′ 9″	142-151	148-160	155-176
5′ 10″	144-154	151-163	158-180
5′ 11″	146-157	154-166	161-184
6′ 0″	149-160	157-170	164-188
6′ 1″	152-164	160-174	168-192
6′ 2″	155-168	164-178	172-197
6′ 3″	158-172	167-182	176-202
6′ 4″	162-176	171-187	181-207

Weights at ages 25-59 based on lowest mortality. Weight in pounds according to frame (in indoor clothing weighing 5 lbs.; shoes with 1″ heels).

If you are anxious, don't be. Losing as little as 5 percent of your body weight helps. Just remember that slow and steady weight loss is the healthy way to lose it for life. No crash diets, starving yourself, or dropping weight too fast. The goal is to make changes that will last. And please, don't ignore the signs and symptoms your physical body may be telling you. Live in the reality that extra weight puts you more at risk for health problems. There is no better reason to lose those extra pounds. Pay attention to your body. It's the only one you have this side of heaven!

PART TWO

CHANGING HOW YOU THINK, FEEL, AND LIVE

God loves you just the way you are,
but he refuses to leave you that way.

— MAX LUCADO

5
Nutrition Transformed!

"You are what you eat!" Hopefully not, or today I would be soup, which would make me warm, delicious, and filling. The good news? There is a more scientific approach to the subject of food and what it does for us. Our LIFL goal is to transform your ho-hum style or habit of eating what may or may not be good for you into a keen awareness and appreciation of why you eat, what you eat, how you eat, and whether you enjoy what goes into your mouth. The transformation will likely make you feel better and also result in a healthier lifestyle.

The first step is to peruse your food journal from Appendix A. If you have not yet tried this exercise, it isn't too late. If you were to start a journal today and follow through for just three days, you would see patterns begin to emerge that point to the decisions you make about the food you eat. So start today!

Your journal provides specifics about your food choices and how much of those foods you eat. As you read through your journal, you will undoubtedly note food choices that are not healthy and need attention. For example, if you see that you usually have a high-calorie sugar snack (such as a donut) around 2:00 p.m. each day, target that snack-time. By substituting a lower-calorie, nutritious snack such as low fat yogurt, for example, you have made a significant change, because small changes implemented daily make a BIG difference over time.

One of my (Steve's) old eating patterns that needed attention was my frequent morning stops at McDonald's™ for breakfast. Almost every day I used to start my day with one or more Egg McMuffins™ (with a lot of jam on the side) and a large soft drink. The surge of sugar, caffeine, cholesterol, grease, and over 1,500 calories ruined any hopes I had of healthy living. Added to that was a fried fruit pie around 10:00 a.m.

I didn't change overnight. But I recognized that I could make a huge impact by changing even one aspect of my eating habit. So I stopped drinking soft drinks and started drinking tea. That slight change alone eliminated hundreds of calories each day. Switching beverages also helped keep my blood sugar more stable, which lowered my cravings. I stopped going to McDonald's™ altogether and started eating eggs and tomatoes or peanut butter on toast with a glass of non-fat milk. The impact of this change was huge. I felt better and the weight began to come down just from that one change. If you have some poor eating habits, changing only one of them can have dramatic impact. In truth, the worse your eating habits are, the more material you have to work with in making small changes that produce big impact.

You don't have to count calories specifically to lose it for life. You will lose weight if you only cut back on calories. For example, if you cut back on just 100 calories a day (such as saying no to a cookie or a third of a candy bar), you would lose approximately ten pounds in a year's time, which can be a big difference! Reducing your portion size and making smarter food choices are two of the easiest and most painless methods to cut calories. Also helpful is to understand the basics about how your body uses food. If you are more comfortable with a complete plan, we provide two possibilities: The Smart Low Carb Weight-Loss Plan and The Walker's Weight-Loss Plan (see Appendix D).

Rising to the Challenge

Four separate verbs make up our overall strategy for healthy eating: reduce, increase, substitute, and eliminate, forming the acronym RISE. And isn't it interesting that the reason we have hope and can overcome difficulties is because of a *risen* Savior? Jesus rose above every challenge and struggle He faced. Even death could not stop Him—He is risen and sits at the right hand of the Father! This fact alone encourages us to an eternal hope and power to live daily in His victory.

REDUCE: white sugar and flour; white rice; potatoes—any and all white processed starches and fat, also refined carbohydrates.

INCREASE: vegetables, lean meats, and fruits low in carbs and high in fiber.

SUBSTITUTE: healthy foods for empty calories and poor nutritional foods .

ELIMINATE: junk food and trans fat.

Reduce

Sugar and Refined Carbohydrates

When there is too much of it, sugar turns to fat! Here's the general idea behind reducing sugar and simple or refined carbohydrates. Our bodies need sugar to function. All carbohydrates contain sugar. However, sugar exists in different forms, some of which are easier to digest than others. The faster sugar is absorbed into the body, the more insulin is produced, creating a rise in blood sugar. *Insulin* is the hormone responsible for circulating sugar into the bloodstream to either be used by organs now or stored for later use. So your body takes the sugar from carbohydrates and converts it to fuel that, when stored, is called "body fat." The more fuel you have stored, the more body fat you have!

Generally speaking, the more food is processed, the faster it is absorbed. When sugars and starches are absorbed quickly into your blood-stream, it is easy to become overweight. Sugar and refined carbohydrates cause rapid changes in blood sugar because they are absorbed quickly. They also stimulate hunger, which may entice you to eat more often.

Our goal is to eat more foods that cause a gradual rise in blood sugar and avoid those that cause blood sugar to spike quickly. One way to become familiar with which foods are healthy regarding sugar is to look at a resource index. In the 1970s, Dr. David Jenkins introduced a new way of categorizing foods—the Glycemic Index (GI), which measures carbohydrates in foods on a scale from 0-100, according to the amount blood sugar rises after eating the food. The lower the score, the longer it takes that food to raise your blood sugar. Therefore, you want to choose foods that are low on the glycemic index. Appendix C lists the glycemic index for a number of foods.

When you significantly reduce or even eliminate high-glycemic foods, you will increase your chances to lose weight. Numerous studies show the significance of the GI in weight control. Low-glycemic foods:

· satisfy your hunger longer, minimize your food cravings better, and help you lose weight.

· result in a lower rise in blood sugar levels after eating and improve diabetes control.

· can enhance your physical endurance and also help refuel carbo-hydrate stores after exercise.

Food choices you can make to lower the glycemic index of your eating plan include choosing breakfast cereals with oats, barley, and bran. Eat breads that are "grainy" with whole seeds—no white bread—and include all types of fruit and vegetables (except potatoes) in your daily menu. Load up on salad vegetables (a vinaigrette dressing is fine) because they have a very low glycemic index count.

Many of us eat high-glycemic carbohydrates in the morning for breakfast (donuts, bagels, white bread toast, and sugary cereals). These carbohydrates may actually make us feel hungrier by midmorning. This idea is being tested and still debated. However, if you find that you are hungry a few hours after breakfast, switch to proteins or a high-fiber cereal and see if it helps.

Fats (Especially the Bad Kind)

Reducing fat should be a part of your meal plan, but it's important to distinguish between the different types of fat. The unsaturated and non-trans fats are the "good" fats. They include olive, canola, and peanut oil, and omega-3 polyunsaturated fat that is found in fish and fish oil capsules. These fats are actually beneficial in a diet in that they help prevent heart disease and stroke. Read food labels and try to stay within the range of no more than 25 percent of your calories coming from fat. You want to cut back on the trans fats, which will be covered in more detail under the "Eliminate" section.

Increase

Fiber

Fiber is the indigestible portion of plant food. It is also an important aid in losing weight because it works to slow the absorption of sugar. It is found mostly in fresh fruits and vegetables, whole grains, and legumes. Fiber slows down digestion and leads to feeling satisfied longer and also decreases appetite. Since we can't digest fiber, the bulk it provides makes you feel full.

Choose high-fiber foods over low-fiber foods. There are any number of high-fiber multigrain breakfast cereals available, not to mention barley, whole wheat bread, and fruits such as pears and raspberries. Eat four servings a week of legumes such as beans, peas, and lentils. Good ways to get these servings include bean or lentil salad, vegetable chili, low-fat refried beans, baked beans, or bean burritos. All it takes to get the recommended dose of fiber daily (20-35 grams) is adding an apple, orange, or one cup of lentils to your meal plan.[27]

Another way to look at this is to eat "big" food. Big food means eating food that has the most volume (nutritional value) with the least amount of calories and carbs. A piece of chocolate cake would be a very "small" food. It has a lot of fat, sugar, calories, and carbs, but very little volume (nutritional value). You can have your cake and eat it too, but it will help if the rest of the day you are eating nutritious, big foods with much larger volumes.

Fill Up and Chill Out

Are you getting enough water? One way to know is to check whether you have any of these symptoms: bad breath, pasty mouth or tongue, intestinal cramping, dark-colored or smelly urine, difficult bowel movements, dry skin, or headaches. If so, add more water to your daily eating plan.

Include hydrating liquids that are nonalcoholic, non-caffeinated, and non-carbonated, such as water, herbal teas, soy or rice drinks (watch the sugar content in these!), and nonfat milk. Alcohol, caffeinated drinks, and carbonated beverages actually dehydrate the body. Drink a 1:1 ratio of water for each of these types of beverages you consume, or simply replace these drinks with water or another hydrating liquid. If you stopped drinking regular soda, for instance, in favor of water, you would reduce sugar and calories by 140-150 calories each time. That small change can add up to about fifteen pounds a year!

We recommend you obtain a favorite water bottle. Fill it with water and keep it with you as a continual reminder to keep on drinking! You may also want to drink an additional glass of water before meals in order to curb your appetite.

If you have difficulty getting in enough water, here is a schedule for drinking water throughout the day that may help:

Begin your day	12 ounces of water
Before lunch	12 ounces of water
After lunch	12 ounces of water
Right before dinner	12 ounces of water
After dinner (but 2 hours before bedtime)	12 ounces of water

Here's a great tip about drinking cold water. Your body needs to warm up cold liquids in order to maintain an internal body temperature, and this process of warming liquids burns calories. According to Jay T. Kearney, former director of sports science and the technology division at the U.S. Olympic Training Center, drinking eight glasses of ice water a day burns about sixty calories.[28] So chill out and fill up!

Dairy

There is good news when it comes to increasing low-fat and non-fat dairy foods in your diet. Foods like hard cheese, yogurt, and milk (consumed in moderation) appear to speed up your metabolism. According to researcher Michael Zemel, calcium found in dairy foods plays a key role in weight loss. When calcium is in the blood, it signals fat cells to stop storing fat and burn it.[29] Therefore, including four low-fat dairy servings a day is a good idea for weight loss and building strong bones. Again, our recommendation is that you make your dairy choices low-fat. Typically we don't recommend this strategy for other foods because low-fat, processed foods are such because they replace fat with carbohydrates. But when it comes to dairy, low-fat is best.

Substitute

Obviously you want to substitute low-fat, healthy foods for high-fat foods of little nutritional value, and low-glycemic foods for higher ones. For example, substitute low-fat, fruit-flavored yogurt for a cinnamon bagel, a cup of sliced cantaloupe for dried apricots (dried fruits are high in sugar), vegetables and low-calorie dip for potato chips and dip, and a bean burrito in a whole wheat tortilla wrap for a beef burrito.

And it's a good idea to try new foods. Our tastes change as we age. There may be food items you never liked as a child that you may enjoy as an adult. For many people, broccoli is one of those foods. Those vegetables you didn't like as a kid often prove to be good adult choices because they are low in fat and low on the glycemic index.

Food substitution is especially important in maintaining weight loss. The best blueberry muffins in my (Steve's) town became a great midmorning snack when I moved to Laguna Beach. But my weight began creeping up almost immediately with that new little habit. Substituting a blueberry bagel for the muffin eliminated fat and sugar and proved satisfying. Sugar-free ice cream hits the spot when I want something cold and sweet. Mustard on turkey sandwiches replaced mayonnaise until I discovered a reduced-fat mayonnaise that I liked. There are so many substitutes on the market for the poor choices that we gradually turn into habits.

Eliminate

Trans fat

As you already know, fats and proteins slow down sugar absorption. Yet not all fats are the same. One type of fat is downright dangerous, so try to eliminate it as much as possible: "trans fat" or trans-fatty acid. Trans-fatty acid is created when hydrogen is bubbled through oil to produce a margarine that doesn't melt at room temperature. Adding trans fat to a food increases its shelf life and often gives food a good flavor.[30] However, trans fat contributes to obesity, a weakened immune system, diabetes, and coronary heart disease because it raises bad cholesterol and blood fats. It also may promote muscle loss and increase your risk for cancer.[31]

Did you know that about 40 percent of the food on grocery store shelves contains partially hydrogenated vegetable oils, which contain trans-fatty acid? (Fortunately there are stores like Wild Oats™ that won't carry a product if it has hydrogenated fat in it!) In the past, these fats have not had to be listed on many products, but the Food and Drug Administration will require trans fat to be listed below the saturated fat line of a product beginning January 1, 2006.[32] Since trans fat is so unhealthy, there are no safe recommended upper limits of consumption. The best strategy is to eliminate it whenever you can.

In the meantime, how do you check food labels? First, look at the ingredient list of a product. The higher up in the list that you see the words "hydrogenated" or "partially hydrogenated," the more trans fat the food contains. So pick foods where it is lower in the list or not there at all. Organic food is better than processed food. Make small choices, such as switching to low-fat milk instead of nondairy creamer in your coffee, or using olive oil, sesame oil, or butter-flavored spray instead of margarine. And choose baked chips over those that are fried. Be creative and take small steps when making these changes. Keep in mind that every poor eating habit you change is helping your overall picture of health.

One important note: There is a distant cousin of trans fat called CLA (conjugated linoleic acid) that naturally occurs in dairy and beef. It is not related to partially hydrogenated oils but is similar in structure. New studies show that CLA may actually be helpful in fighting off the very thing its cousin brings about.[33]

Menu Recommendations

Healthy eating can be greatly helped with the addition of a menu of good, tasty food choices. Here are a few suggestions to get started:

Breakfast

Eat an energy-building breakfast that gives you a good start for the day! Make it a priority to eat some protein as it will help to curb your hunger between meals. When using milk, consider using a lower fat percentage grade milk or even skim milk. And when making pancakes or waffles, consider using low or no-fat yogurt or buttermilk.

Also consider adding fruit and whole wheat flour to pancake or muffin mixes. Fruit is a great addition to whole-grain cereals too. Also, eggs are fine to eat for breakfast, when eaten in moderation. Make omelets or scrambled eggs by using Egg Beaters™ or egg whites. Throw in some diced vegetables for a tasty breakfast.

Lunch

Make the usual turkey on whole-grain bread more exciting by adding cut up red peppers and a couple of pea pods for nutrients. Eliminate or reduce the mayonnaise altogether and opt instead for mustard or Lemonaise Lite™. Try to squeeze in more veggies to your daily menu by eating a spinach salad. Rediscover soup—healthy soup, that is! Though it takes time to eat, the fact that you are slowed down may help to keep you from overeating.

Dinner

Eat fish a couple of times a week, especially albacore tuna and salmon. Consider having a vegetarian meal one or two nights a week as well. If you are new to vegetarian cooking, try stir-frying some veggies with tofu in sesame oil; or cook up whole-wheat spaghetti with peas and chopped tomatoes and sprinkle with low-fat or soy parmesan cheese.

When eating meat, try meat strips in place of a full cut of meat. Use sliced beef or chicken to make fajitas by grilling marinated meat with onions, peppers, and tomatoes. Or consider making shish kabobs by cutting up meat or chunks of fish alongside fruit or vegetable chunks. Broil or grill the kabobs and serve with brown rice.

Snacks

A cup of strawberries meets your quota for two servings of fruit and provides all the vitamin C needs for a day. Blueberries are loaded with antioxidants and contain a compound called pterostilbene, which may even lower your cholesterol. And there is a reason why an apple a day keeps the doctor away—it is nature's perfect fruit! You should eat one to two apples every day.

Designing Your Own Meal Plan

To lose weight, your goal is to burn more calories a day than you eat. You can design your own plan tailored to your likes and dislikes or choose instead one of the two plans we have provided.

Calorie Count

Whichever plan you choose, the first step is to determine your current calorie intake. Here's an easy way to find out that number. First, decide how active you are. *Sedentary* means you have a job or lifestyle that involves mostly sitting, standing, or light walking; you exercise once a week. *Active* means your job or lifestyle requires more activity than light walking (such as full-time housecleaning or construction work), or you get forty-five to sixty minutes of aerobic exercise three times a week. *Very Active* means you get aerobic exercise for at least forty-five to sixty minutes four or more times a week.

Choose the description that best fits your current lifestyle, and then locate your activity factor from the table below:

You Are a:	Your Factor Is:
Sedentary woman	12
Sedentary man	14
Active woman	15
Active man	17
Very active woman	18
Very active man	20

Next, multiply your activity factor by your current weight in pounds. The resulting number is the approximate number of calories you need to maintain your current weight. An example for an active woman who weighs 150 pounds would look like this: *15 x 150 = 2,250 calories*. So if this 150-pound woman wanted to lose weight, she would need to restrict her calorie intake to less than 2,250 calories.

If you prefer to not be on a strict plan but want to watch labels instead, we recommend simply reducing your current calorie intake by 500-1,000 calories each day. This will lead to safe, effective weight loss of one to two pounds per week. Please note that you should *never* go below 1,500 calories per day unless under the supervision of a doctor.

Two Personal Plans

Included in this book are two weight loss plans: The Smart Low-Carb Plan and The Walker's Plan. For both plans, consult the following chart to plan meals; it's important to eat the number of servings listed for each food group. Appendix D includes meal plans and recipes for both plans.

The average diet is full of carbohydrates that take up an estimated

50 to 60 percent of the total number of calories consumed. Based on the calorie level you just calculated, check the table below to find out the approximate number of grams of carbohydrates in your current diet. You might be surprised by the number. This table assumes that 55 percent of the calories in your diet come from carbohydrates, but if your diet is more heavily weighted in carbohydrates, these figures may even be on the low side.

Daily Calories	Carbs (grams)
1800	248
2000	275
2400	330
2800	385

If you feel you are cutting back carbohydrates too soon, eat 180 grams a day instead of 125. Stay on this schedule for several weeks before switching to 125 grams a day. Most people who consume a low-fat diet will likely lose weight by cutting their carbohydrate intake to 125 grams daily.

Handling Cravings

Sugar

Have you ever said, "I'm addicted to sugar"? Well, you may not be too far from the truth. New studies (mostly in animals) show that a habit of overeating sweets may share some characteristics of serious addictions.[34] There is no direct proof as of yet, but the theory involves the activation of natural opioids in the brain. There is enough similarity that researchers are studying the connection between cravings and brain chemistry.

Dr. Bart Hoebel, a psychologist at Princeton University who conducts animal studies, reports, "People with a genetic predisposition for addiction can become overly dependent on sugar, particularly if they periodically stop eating and then binge." His research indicates that abstinence can bring about withdrawal symptoms similar to drug addiction. "The taste of sugar makes the brain release natural opioids, and the bingeing causes dopamine release." While sugar cravings are yet to be understood, there is possibly some connection to brain chemistry and dependency. According to Dr. Braly, medical director of York Nutritional Laboratories and author of *Food Allergy Relief,* "People with food cravings may actually have neurochemical and hormonal imbalances that trigger these cravings."[35]

While the jury is still out as to whether sugar is truly addictive, one way to circumvent the problem is to simply avoid sugar altogether or find a way to deal with cravings. Distraction is a good answer. If you remove yourself from a situation in which sugary foods are available and wait forty-five minutes to an hour, the craving will probably go away. If you are still thinking about a food item after that much time, have a small amount of it. Other ways to distract yourself are to use physical exercise, relaxation exercises like deep breathing, or involvement in a new activity such as reading.

For some people, there is little question that sugar is addictive. Perhaps the best alternative, if you cannot stop with a small treat, is to forego the treat altogether. Sugar is not a food group we have to have. This is a hard journey to travel and you will have to resolve potential feelings of deprivation, but it may be the only way you can succeed at long-term weight loss.

Chocolate

Give me chocolate or give me death! People crave chocolate more than any other food. Research investigating both the physiological and psychological basis of chocolate cravings remains inconclusive. It is most likely a combination of both. If you are going to eat chocolate, eat small amounts and choose dark chocolate because it has less sugar and fat. Apparently the cocoa in dark chocolate, a plant derivative, has been shown to have antioxidant benefits.[36] However, a little goes a long way because chocolate is calorie dense.

Changing Your Behavior

Eat Breakfast

We can't tell you how many people think losing weight is about skipping breakfast. And they couldn't be more wrong if they tried! A wealth of research supports the fact that eating breakfast is key to losing weight and maintaining a healthy lifestyle. Eating breakfast:

- has been linked to having a lower body mass, compared to people who skip the meal.
- reduces a person's risk of obesity and insulin resistance.
- is a proven strategy to maintaining long-term weight loss.
- improves grades and behavior among school children.[37]

Weigh Yourself Regularly

Weigh yourself daily? No way! It sounds counterintuitive, but the members of the National Weight Control Registry, a group of over 4,500 successful dieters who have lost at least thirty pounds and kept it off for at least one year, say weighing regularly helps keep the weight off.[38] Weekly weigh-ins are characteristic of 75 percent of members, while 44.5 percent weigh daily.

Even though we can usually tell by the fit or looseness of our clothing, the scale is used to self-monitor as a guard against those pounds creeping back without our awareness. Keeping a daily account of your weight will give you the feedback you need to cut back or maintain your weight. Once you notice a three- to five-pound weight gain, it's time to cut back and increase your exercise. Remember, if you overeat at one meal, you can cut back on the next meal.

Every new day is a chance to start afresh. As we are reminded in Lamentations 3:22-24 (MSG), "GOD's loyal love couldn't have run out, his merciful love couldn't have dried up. They're created new every morning. How great your faithfulness! I'm sticking with GOD (I say it over and over). He's all I've got left." We need to apply His "new mercies" to our lives daily and walk in victory.

Control Portions

Sizes have really increased in the last few years. Just think about fast food chains. Nearly everything you buy can be super-sized for just a few pennies more. And foods that don't appear in multiples can also be sized too big for one serving. For example, one Noah's™ bagel constitutes four servings from the bread group. Next time you order pasta in a restaurant, look to see if the portion size is about half a cup (one serving). Most likely, you'll be served three or more cups (six serving sizes). And most people clean their plates in restaurants—after all, they've paid for the food!

According to nutrition researcher Lisa Young of New York State University, portions are about twice as large as they were twenty years ago.[39] So downsize your orders, share an entrée when dining out, and pay attention to the amount of food you eat.

Keep in mind, however, that it is a mistake to reduce your portions to the point that you feel deprived or even hungry at the end of a meal. Instead, the solution is to eat more foods that have a lower-calorie density and a high volume of nutrition. Change out small-volume foods for big-volume foods. You won't pack on the weight if you load up on veggies and low-calorie soups, but you will feel full!

Replace a Meal

Here's a tip you may want to try from time to time. Replace one of your meals with a portion-controlled food or commercial liquid diet drink. If you aren't sure how much you've been overeating, use a meal substitute for a lunch to bring yourself back under control. A meal replacement tells you exactly how many calories you are getting and so there is no guess work to do. Just eat or drink up and get back on your regular plan.

Eat More Often

Gently changing *how* you eat produces a positive effect on *what* you eat. Be sure to eat an energy-building breakfast that gets you off to a good start! Eat more meals throughout the day without changing the amount of calories you are taking in. If you eat six mini meals a day, you don't have to pack in the food in order to "make it" until the next meal four hours later. Instead, eat smaller meals every two hours. In fact, research supports the fact that people who eat smaller, frequent meals are thinner and healthier.[40]

Don't Go Hungry to an Event

If you know you are going to an event like an office party, buffet party, or a celebration such as a wedding, don't go hungry. You will overeat, guaranteed. Instead, plan ahead. Drink a full glass of water and eat a piece of fruit before you leave; this small action will curb your appetite and help you resist the goodies you encounter. Place yourself next to a low-calorie snack if you have the munchies. And if you are asked to bring a food or dish, make it a vegetable tray or some other healthy choice that you can nibble on throughout the event.

Routine Is Good

One of the most common problems encountered when trying to lose weight is dealing with all the food choices available. The more variety you have to choose from, the more likely you will be to overeat. Research bears this out.[41] Establishing an eating routine helps. You don't have to be boring and eat the exact same thing each day, but monotony and following a basic schedule of what to eat does help people stick to their plans.

Don't Cook Foods You Have Trouble Resisting

When you are trying to lose weight, don't cook or bake foods you are tempted to eat. Your family will understand and can live without Mom's famous German chocolate cake! Sometimes we feel guilty "depriving" others of the goodies we have decided to forego. We shouldn't. Lose the guilt and focus on the fact that our decision to lose weight is helping the family make changes for the better as well. No one will suffer from the absence of fudge brownies for dessert. Trust us; it won't come up in therapy twenty years from now!

Variety May Not Be the Spice of Life

In a recent study,[42] Brian Wansink, a professor of marketing and nutritional science at the University of Illinois at Urbana-Champaign, gives support to the idea that more than willpower is involved in resisting food. The color of food, the way it is displayed, and a person's perception of variety can lead to overeating. He says, "People eat more with their eyes, and their eyes trick their stomachs." Based on his study, he offers these tips to prevent unhealthy overeating:

1. Multiple bowls of the same food give you the perception that there is more variety. Therefore, at parties, avoid multiple bowls.

2. At a buffet or reception, don't have more than two different foods on your plate at a time. In fact, decrease the variety of foods on your plate as much as possible.

3. If you arrange fruits and vegetables on your plate in an unorganized fashion, it will stimulate your appetite.

Create a Safe Eating Environment

It's very important to create an eating atmosphere that is free of anxiety. Mealtime should be enjoyable and relaxing. Unfortunately, this wasn't the case in many of your homes growing up. But now, as an adult, you can take charge of meals and make them pleasant. Engage in pleasant conversation, have soft music playing in the background, or light candles. Make mealtime an "up" part of the day. If you eat alone, make your place setting attractive. Enjoy the quiet and concentrate on taking your time and relaxing. Chewing food slowly and eating without rushing will help you savor your food. Proverbs 23:2-3 tells us, "Don't gobble your food, don't talk with your mouth full. And don't stuff yourself; bridle your appetite" (MSG).

You should establish regular mealtimes and eat them at the kitchen or dining room table. Eating in front of the TV, on the run, in the car, or while reading a book is a setup for "unconscious" eating. Eating becomes "unconscious" when you hardly remember doing it! It should not be considered an activity to multi-task with. Break the habit of eating in places other than at the table.

Also, make sure you sit down while you eat. This will help break the habit of eating while you cook, clean up, or serve others. A little taste here and there can really add on the pounds. By using the same place settings (pick small plates!), you will establish a routine for your meals. It may be psychological that small plates help us eat less, but it works to trick you into thinking you are getting plenty of food.

Another way to create a safe environment is to rid your house of tempting high-fat foods or binge foods. For example, if you have a hard time resisting Oreo™ cookies, don't buy them. If you are trying not to snack on chips, keep them out of your pantry. You won't be tempted by what is missing, and you will have to eat what is available. So have healthy low-calorie snacks available to munch on for those hungry moments. Go through your pantry and toss out the chips, sodas, and cookies; load up on fruit, nuts, and veggies.

We also advise putting leftovers out of sight right after the meal is over. Don't leave them on the counter. Seal them in foil so you don't look at the food every time you open the refrigerator or freezer door, because when you can't see it, it's less tempting! And remember to distinguish between physical hunger and hunger related to emotions such as boredom or stress. Turn off TV commercials or switch channels when an advertisement gives you a craving. Pass by the magazine food advertisements. There is enough evidence to suggest that looking at pictures of food cues your desire to eat it,[43] so don't look at those pictures!

In addition, you should eat in full view of friends and family. Secret eating gets people in trouble. Sometimes we think that sneaking food or eating in secret doesn't count. But that isn't true, and hiding from the reality only hurts you.

Dining Out

Let's face it. Few of us eat all our meals at home. In our fast-paced lives, dining out is a reality, but it doesn't have to be a nightmare if you are trying to lose weight. Here are ten tips for dining out compiled by Nanci Hellmich of *USA Today* after she talked with four nutritionists[44]:

1. Order less of something. Ask for half a portion or a junior portion of what's served.

2. Choose a sauce that is red versus white or pink. Red sauces are usually tomato-based and have less fat and fewer calories.

3. Skip the breadbasket. Either ask the server not to bring it, to bring it late in the meal, or to only serve one slice of bread.

4. Order soup (broth-based) prior to eating an entrée. It will fill you up.

5. Avoid large portions on the menu and descriptions that sound like trouble, such as "fried," "battered," or "buttery."

6. Order steamed or sautéed vegetables as a side dish.

7. Take half the meal and wrap it up before you even begin to eat it. You won't be tempted to eat past your feelings of fullness if the remainder of the meal isn't on the plate.

8. Split a dessert or only take one bite. If you really want something for yourself, order a cappuccino with (low-fat) milk and add some sugar (or Splenda®). This treat is only about 100 calories!

9. Avoid anything super-sized. Order a kid-sized portion if you can.

10. Instead of an entrée, order an appetizer. The portion size is usually smaller and plenty filling.

Dining in the Sky

Eating meals on an airplane can create a challenge. If you know a meal will be served on a particular flight, you can request a special meal (low-fat, vegetarian, or seafood) if you call ahead and place an order. Also, many hotels will box up food for you to take on a plane. Or you could walk to a local food market and package a meal or snack to take along. Make sure to drink plenty of water, since airplane travel dehydrates travelers. Avoid coffee and alcohol for this reason.

Eating should be a pleasure. And although losing weight means adjusting eating habits and patterns, it does not have to result in out-of-control feelings of deprivation or frustration. The important thing is to choose an eating plan and foods that will improve your energy and health. Follow the RISE formula to do this—it really works! And remember, small changes that you can stick with are much more powerful than big ones you won't continue. So make changes you can live with to establish healthy eating habits that will last for life.

6
Move It *and* Lose It

You've heard the saying, "Move it or lose it!" We'd like to alter it a bit to, "Move it *and* lose it." That's right. The more you move it, the more you'll lose it—or at least keep from going in the opposite direction! Even though exercise will not turn you into Twiggy (for those of you too young to remember, she was a very skinny model from the 1960s), it is responsible for keeping most of us from gaining weight. Members of the National Weight Control Registry report that exercise plays a role in keeping their weight off as well. Most reported exercising about an hour a day.[45]

Okay, so an hour a day sounds like torture to some of you. Not to worry! We are convinced that there is at least one activity you can really enjoy. There isn't a requirement to exercise for sixty minutes straight either. So take a deep breath and relax. Exercise can work for you.

To begin, let's revisit our RISE formula and apply it to exercise.

REDUCE: your negativity and lackadaisical attitude toward exercise.

INCREASE: your physical activity, water consumption, commitment to exercise, and accountability.

SUBSTITUTE: the right attitude—a cheerful one—if need be, and also the right workout clothing for the wrong apparel.

ELIMINATE: all excuses for not exercising! Exercise isn't optional in Lose It For Life.

Steve's Secret

This is the area of Lose It For Life that was the most transforming for me. Before I finally lost the weight for good, I couldn't jog around the block, and I saw no reason to try. I was so out of shape that even walking up a flight of stairs created intense embarrassment for me. I smoked and was fat and just saw no reason to exercise. I admit it; I hated the very idea of exercising. I saw it as something no one in their right mind would engage in regularly because they wanted to. But all that has changed. I am living proof of the transformation that can occur when a person decides to start exercising and sticks with it.

I went jogging this morning before church and had a great run by the water. Once I was finished, I felt so good knowing I had done something for myself and my health. I now view exercise as a gift from God. It not only helps me control my weight and improve my health, but it also improves the quality of my life.

There is one point that I want to stress: If you struggle with exercising, there is a way to make it better that has proven successful over and over again: Find an exercise partner. I have seen people struggle with their weight for decades and then find success because they were held accountable and kept moving. It doesn't cost anything to have a friend who will exercise with you! But it will keep you from turning over and going back to sleep rather than getting up and moving.

If you don't have any friends, or you live in a swamp, or you're in a relationship that won't allow you to have friends, you should know that your excuses are nothing new! So when you are ready, overcome the excuses, get a partner, and realize that you just may have found the key to the long-term weight loss you have been looking for.

Do you absolutely hate the very idea of exercise? Let's take a little quiz and see if you have the right mindset to get moving. (Use the answer key below to see how ready you are to jump in and begin moving, based on the number of times you answered yes.)

Ready to Exercise?

1. Does the very idea of exercise bore you?   Y N

2. Are you a pro at finding excuses not to engage in physical activities?   Y N

3. If a friend invited you to go on a bike ride, would you suggest meeting for lunch instead?   Y N

4. Do you get tired watching someone else work out?   Y N

5. Do you choose the elevator over stairs every chance you get?   Y N

6. Have you given up exercising because you weren't satisfied with previous results?   Y N

7. Are you waiting to lose weight until you start exercising?   Y N

8. Do you hate the idea of breaking a sweat?   Y N

9. Do you resolve to take up exercising year after year but never seem to get around to it?   Y N

10. When you are running errands, do you often drive rather than walk?   Y N

0-2: YOU'RE READY TO REAP THE ENERGY-BOOSTING BENEFITS OF EXERCISE. You're actually pro-exercise, but there may be a few things keeping you from fully adopting an active lifestyle. Revisit a sport you enjoyed in your youth. Or choose something new that you've always wanted to learn or do.

3-5: YOUR FITNESS HURDLES ARE MAINLY ATTITUDE-INDUCED. If you've been unhappy with past exercise efforts, you may have expected results too soon. While exercise often feels good in a matter of days, it usually takes a month to see real cardiovascular and strength benefits. For instant encouragement, keep a graph that shows the length and frequency of your workouts.

6-10: YOU'RE ON THE WRONG SIDE OF THE STARTING GATE. Your excuses for skipping workouts only cheat yourself. When you're tempted to skip, think about this study from the Veterans' Affairs Palo Alto Health Care System at Stanford University: A person's peak exercise capacity, as measured on a treadmill test, is a more powerful predictor of longevity than health risk factors such as heart disease, high blood pressure, or smoking.

How Much Is Enough?

Your attitude toward exercising matters—in fact, it's as important as the food you put in your mouth. Since finding time to exercise is usually a factor for most people who struggle to get moving, consider this. According to the results of a series of studies undertaken at the University of Pittsburgh, women who were told to exercise in ten-minute bouts four times a day exercised more and lost more weight than women told to exercise for forty minutes once a day. Most of the women in the study chose walking for their exercise. Those who exercised in short bouts lost about twenty pounds after twenty-six weeks, while those who exercised in longer stretches lost only about thirteen pounds.[46] This fact should be of great encouragement if you struggle to find significant blocks of time in the day to exercise. You also may benefit from this strategy if you are someone who physically hurts when exercising. If you aren't sure what can be done in just ten minutes, turn to Appendix E for our Ten-Minute Workout.

While the above study encourages you to exercise for short periods throughout the day, more recent recommendations from the Institute of Medicine (IOM) provide a different recommendation. In September of 2002, the IOM recommended that adults engage in sixty minutes of moderate intense physical exercise, such as brisk walking, every day.[47] The time length differs from the U.S. Surgeon General's 1996 recommendation of thirty minutes of daily exercise. The IOM has increased the daily time because of the increased calorie consumption and weight of most Americans. Twenty to thirty minutes of high-intensity daily exercise would meet their guidelines as well. So while this is a bit of a confusing picture, your best bet is to exercise somewhere between thirty and sixty minutes a day.

A quick note regarding your health—since exercise is so important to your overall success, make sure you are physically ready to begin. According to the President's Council on Physical Fitness and Health, if you are under age thirty-five and in good health, you don't have to see a doctor before beginning an exercise program. However, if you are over thirty-five and have been inactive for several years, you should consult with a doctor.[48] If for any reason you aren't sure how to proceed or have questions about your health, ask your doctor if there are any special concerns that need to be faced before you begin.

Benefits of Exercise

There are so many benefits when it comes to exercise. Here are six of the best reasons:

- Exercise helps reduce hidden belly fat, lowering the risk of heart disease, diabetes, stroke, and some types of cancer.[49]

· Exercise prevents muscle from wasting and helps to lose fat.[50]

· Exercise helps the brain deal with stress more effectively.[51]

· Moderate cardiovascular exercise such as thirty minutes of brisk walking a few times a week can improve your memory.[52]

· Exercise helps manage hunger. Research shows that exercising increases control over hunger and food intake. In fact, the physically fit person is often not hungry until several hours after exercise.[53]

· Exercise improves your immune system.[54]

We can't stress this point enough: *When it comes to making exercise a habit, attitude is more than half the battle.* Whatever reasons you have used for avoiding exercise in the past—it's unpleasant, too painful, inconvenient, frustrating, or too time consuming—the reality is that exercise is necessary if you are serious about being healthy. Regardless of your past experiences, regular physical activity is essential for weight control and developing a healthy lifestyle.

Physical activity increases the number of calories your body uses and promotes the loss of body fat instead of muscle and other nonfat tissue. In addition to promoting weight control, physical activity improves your strength and flexibility, lowers your risk of heart disease, helps control blood pressure and diabetes, can promote a sense of well-being, and can decrease stress.[55]

Finally, it is documented truth that the more sedentary you are, the more likely you are to be overweight. So any activity, however small, is a change in the right direction. Remember to appreciate what you can do, even if you think it's a small amount. Moving any part of your body, even for a short time, can add up to a big difference. And being physically active doesn't have to occur only when you are in sweats and working out at the gym. If money is an issue, cost doesn't have to get in the way. There are many free ways to exercise, either by yourself or with friends. You can find a local school track where you can walk or run, or walk around a mall before the stores open. Parks are a great place to walk or jog, and quite often you can find a time of the day when they are empty if you prefer a little more privacy while you exercise.

Consider smaller day-to-day changes to improve your health over dramatic goals and types of exercise that will not last. Try taking short walking breaks at work a few times a day, or marching in place during TV commercials. (Okay, we admit, that could be embarrassing, so be careful you don't do it where they might cart you off under the care of mental health workers in white suits!) Taking the stairs instead of the elevator and walking the dog are also good choices. With the advent of the cellular phone, walking while catching up with old friends you can't be physically near is now possible, even if you are just pacing around the house!

Parking your vehicle far away from the mall entrance so you can walk the extra distance is another relatively painless choice. If you take the bus or subway to work, get off one stop early and walk! One of the less touted but still very healthy forms of exercise is working around the house—whether you mow the lawn (no riding mowers, please), rake leaves, garden, or spring clean, you will be moving!

Matching Exercise with Who You Are

Though you won't be expected to do more than you are capable of doing, exercise is essential to the overall program. Choose activities that mesh well with who you are and what you like to do, and you'll be more likely to stick to them. And if an activity provides mental relaxation and enjoyment, you'll receive double the benefits! The following quiz will help you identify what activities are a good match for you, based on your personality, workout goals, and schedule. By combining the results of the three parts of this quiz, you'll have figured out your total fitness personality.[56]

What Is My Personality?

Part One: My Personality and Hobbies
(Circle the letter that most represents you.)

1. As a kid, the activities I liked best were:

   a. gymnastics, cheerleading, jump rope, or dance classes.

   b. playing outside—such as building forts or lemonade stands, climbing trees, exploring the woods, etc.

   c. competitive sports.

   d. playing with dolls, reading, coloring, or art projects.

   e. parties, playing with my friends.

2. My favorite hobbies today are:

   a. anything new and challenging.

   b. outside activities—gardening, walking the dog, watching the stars.

   c. tennis, card or board games, team and/or spectator sports.

   d. reading, movies, needle crafts, painting, or anything that provides an escape.

   e. group activities with friends—anything from a walking club, joining a book group, to just talking.

3. I get motivated to exercise if:

   a. I get a new exercise video or piece of equipment, or I try a totally new fitness class.

   b. I get a new piece of outside equipment, I discover a new walking or jogging path, or the weather is nice.

   c. I'm presented with some competition.

   d. I find an exercise that I get into to the point that I forget my surroundings.

   e. I exercise in a group.

4. I prefer to exercise:

   a. indoors.

   b. outdoors.

   c. wherever there's a competition.

   d. wherever I am not the center of attention.

   e. in a gym or fitness center, not at home.

Interpreting Your Score (Part One)

If you circled mostly the letter "a" or there is not an emerging pattern within your choices, you are probably the Learner. You're always trying something new and welcome physical and mental challenges. You are most likely an "associative exerciser," meaning you focus on the way your body moves and feels when you exercise. Choose activities that help you explore new moves: aerobics classes, any form of dance, Pilates, seated aerobics, inline skating, skipping rope, fencing, or any other activity that attracts your interest.

If you circled mostly the letter "b," you would be classified as an Outdoors Person. Fresh air is your energizer. So why not include nature in your exercise routine? Try hiking, biking, nature walking, gardening, swimming laps, or cross-country skiing.

If you circled mostly the letter "c," you are classified as the Competitor. You naturally like one-on-one, competitive types of activities. Try fencing, cardio kickboxing, and spinning classes. If you excelled in or enjoyed a sport when you were younger, take it up again.

If you circled mostly the letter "d," you are classified as Timid. You're a "disassociative exerciser," meaning you fantasize or think of events in your life when you exercise rather than contemplating the exercise itself. You're more like a wallflower than a participant.

You'll like mind/body activities like Pilates and stretching. Also try nature walking or hiking. You'll also probably love exercise classes. Sign up for classes such as aerobics, cardio kickboxing, seated aerobics, spinning, step aerobics, or water aerobics.

If you circled mostly the letter "e," you are classified as a Social Butterfly. As a people-person, you tend to prefer the gym to exercising in your living room. Try aerobics classes, kickboxing, seated aerobics, spinning classes, stretching, step aerobics, and water aerobics. For weight lifting, find a buddy or two and do circuit training.

Part Two: My Workout Style and Goals

(Circle the letter that most represents you.)

1. My primary exercise goal is:

   a. to lose weight or tone up.

   b. to relax and relieve stress.

   c. to have fun.

   d. depends on how I feel.

2. I prefer:

   a. a lot of structure in my workout.

   b. some structure, but not too much.

   c. no structure.

   d. depends on my mood.

3. I prefer to exercise:

   a. alone.

   b. with one other person.

   c. in a group.

   d. depends on my mood.

Interpreting Your Score (Part Two)

If you circled mostly the letter "a" or a mixture of letters, you're classified as a Gung-ho Exerciser. You don't mess around when you work out. You're there to lose weight and tone up—period. You'll benefit most from doing a specific activity, like cycling, aerobics, or using an elliptical machine, treadmill, or stair climber, at a moderate intensity. For optimal weight loss benefits, you should burn 2,000 calories a week. One way to achieve this would be to perform thirty minutes of aerobic-based exercise daily, combined with three sessions of weight training per week.

If you circled mostly the letter "b," you would be classified as a Leisurely Exerciser. Your main exercise objectives are to relax and de-stress. To relax, try stretching. Studies have shown a direct relationship between physical activity and stress reduction. Hop on the treadmill or head outside and walk for five minutes, run slowly for thirty seconds, and then run fast for thirty seconds, repeating this sequence for about thirty minutes. Circuit weight training is another great interval workout. You do all your reps, then you rest, then you do a few more, and then you rest.

If you circled mostly the letter "c," you are classified as a Fun-Loving Exerciser. Fifty straight minutes on the treadmill is not your bag—there's no room in your fun-filled life. You'll be most likely to stick to activities that are already an integral part of your schedule. Grab your inline skates and circle the neighborhood. Put on your favorite music CD and dance around the living room. And you can make your weight routine more amusing by doing circuit weight training.

If you circled mostly the letter "d," you are classified as a Flexible Exerciser. Exercise turns you on, but routine doesn't. You'd rather fly by the seat of your gym shorts, which is fine. To add variety, use the elliptical machine one day, the treadmill the next, and the cross-country skiing machine the next.

Part Three: My Lifestyle and Schedule

(Circle the letter that most represents you.)

1. I have the most energy:
   a. in the morning.
   b. in the middle of the day.
   c. in the evening or at night.
   d. my energy level fluctuates.

2. I have the most time:
   a. in the morning.
   b. in the middle of the day.
   c. in the evening.
   d. depends on the day.

3. I'm most likely to:
   a. go to bed early and get up early.
   b. go to bed and get up at the same time every day, but not particularly early or late.
   c. go to bed late and get up late.
   d. depends on the day.

Interpreting Your Score (Part Three)

If you circled mostly the letter "a" or a mixture of letters, you're classified as a Morning Dove. You like to get chores out of the way as soon as you get up because that's when you have the most energy. Whether you go to the gym before you start your day or head outside for a dawn walk, you'll have an extra edge over those who hit the snooze button a few more times.

If you circled mostly the letter "b," you would be classified as a Midday Duck. You'd rather plop down on an exercise bike than in front of a sandwich when noon rolls around. Whether you're at home or work, exercise is a great way to break up your day.

If you circled mostly the letter "c," you are classified as a Night Owl. You haven't seen a sunrise since that all-night party in 1974. If you have more energy at night, use that time to exercise. Just don't do it too close to bedtime, or you'll have trouble sleeping.

If you circled mostly the letter "d," you are classified as a Flexible Bird. The best time of day for you to exercise varies with your schedule. So just go with it and don't try and set yourself up with an intense schedule. But do push yourself to exercise as often as possible!

Safety Tips

Drink Plenty of Water

Whenever you exercise, make hydrating your body a priority. Water is beneficial to every cell and organ in your body. It cushions your joints, improves your bowel functions, and keeps your body cool. Drink it before, during, and after exercise.

Pay Attention to Your Body During Exercise

If you become out of breath while exercising, slow down. You should be able to talk while you exercise and not be gasping for air. Do not ignore pain or discomfort when you exercise, as you could do harm to your body. If you notice any of the following signs,[57] stop exercising immediately and contact your health care provider:

· Shortness of breath

· Pain or pressure in the mid-chest area, left side of your neck, left shoulder, or left arm

· Dizziness or nausea

· Break out in a cold sweat

· Muscle cramps or pain in your joints, feet, ankles, or legs

Wear Appropriate Clothing

When you exercise, it helps to wear clothes that are lightweight and loose-fitting so you can move easily. Wear supportive athletic shoes for weight-bearing activities. And when your shoes need to be replaced, don't put it off. If you are a woman, a good support bra is an essential piece of workout equipment. For all clothing, choose fabrics that absorb sweat and remove it from the skin. Never wear rubber or plastic suits, as these could hold the sweat on your skin and make your body overheat.

When exercising outdoors, wear a knit hat to keep you warm in cold weather. A baseball cap is a good choice when the weather is hot in order to shade your face and keep you cool. And don't forget the sunscreen when you venture outside!

It Gets Easier with Time

If you still feel a bit overwhelmed by adding exercise to your daily routine, this journal entry from Cathy may motivate you. She hated to exercise. It hurt! And the embarrassment was almost too much to bear, but she really wanted to lose it for life.

I am down to 272. That is 78 pounds gone forever! I am doing a lot better on my softball team. I am the catcher. About a month ago, I could barely squat down to catch the pitch. And once I was down, I hated to have to stand back up. I actually got dizzy and saw stars because I was so out of shape. I would basically stay down unless I absolutely had to get up to get the ball.

Things have definitely changed for the better! I played a double-header last Thursday night and another doubleheader on Friday. I can now squat down for every pitch, and I quickly stand back up to throw the ball back to the pitcher. I love it! I feel like a regular person, athletic and all! I received comments and hugs from the other players—they said I was the best catcher Crossroads has ever had, and they said they're proud of me for sticking with it.

The First Step

Consistent exercise will take commitment. Don't be afraid of that word, however. You can do this with God's help and the help of others. Success is at the end of many tasks like healthy eating, getting enough sleep, and spending time with the Lord each day. Boundaries and accountability are necessary.

We take care of ourselves by setting boundaries with our time and energy so that there is time for the priorities such as healthy eating and exercising. Decide that your fitness, nutrition, spiritual, and personal time is non-negotiable. This means exercising should not be the first thing you take out of your schedule if life's "stuff" gets in the way. Make every effort to stay with your routine. There is grace for those times when we allow life to crowd out our personal commitments, but we must make it a priority to get back on track and make time for exercise.

If you do not carve out time for your physical, spiritual, and personal needs, you will burn out, bum out, and bail out by acting out. Over-

Check Your Heart Rate

Pace yourself. Remember to slow down if you're too out of breath to carry on a conversation. Before you begin, you should know how to take your heart rate. It's a great measure of intensity during aerobic exercise.

Your resting heart rate can be taken after sitting quietly for five minutes. Count your pulse for 10 seconds and multiply that number by six to get your heart's per-minute rate. For example, if your resting heart rate for 10 seconds is 13 beats, your heart's per-minute rate is 78 (13 x 6 = 78). When you exercise, check your pulse rate five seconds after interrupting your activity. Your target heart rate is calculated by taking the maximum heart rate and multiplying it by 70 percent. Your maximum heart rate is figured by taking 220 minus your age.[58] For example, if you are 40 years old, your maximum heart rate is 180 (220 – 40 = 180). Then multiply 180 by 70% to arrive at your target heart rate of 126 beats per minute (180 x 70% = 126). In order to really benefit from exercising, you should raise your heart rate and sustain it at your target heart rate for 12-15 minutes. So, if you're 40 years old, you should exercise in a manner that will keep your heart rate at 126 beats per minute for 12-15 minutes. The goal is to maintain 55-85 percent of your maximum heart rate for 20-60 minutes.

The more intense the workout, the shorter it needs to be (but not less than 20 minutes).

eating, overworking, drinking, anger, depression, worry, and anxiety are all symptoms of "burnout." Create good habits and routines for exercise, nutrition, and spiritual and personal time so you won't burn out.

If you find yourself unable to exercise consistently, you need more accountability! Find someone who has the discipline you're lacking and ask him/her to help you. Draw help from this person and make the most of their presence and encouragement to provide the structure you need until you are able to provide it for yourself. As you begin a new exercise program, start slowly. Your body needs time to get used to your new activity. Fitness doesn't happen overnight. Be patient and give the process time to work.

We suggest setting short- and long-term goals for your exercise routine. If you have difficulty exercising, a good short-term goal may be to walk for five minutes at least two days per week for two weeks. A long-term goal may be to walk forty minutes most days of the week after nine months. Writing down your progress in a journal is an excellent way to track goals and stay on track. Though you may not feel like you are making progress within a given week, when you look back at where you started, you may be pleasantly surprised!

As was stressed earlier, support is a key factor in staying motivated. An exercise buddy can cheer you on and hold you accountable. For women in particular, it's a good way to feel safe while exercising outdoors.

Establish a Routine

The goal is to find whatever is necessary—tools, books, therapists, or personal trainers—to help you establish a routine you can do for the rest of your life. If you approach a routine with this mindset, finding a pace that is workable will be easier and you will be more likely to stick with it. Don't give up if you miss a few days. Just pick up where you left off and jump right back into the routine.

Five Keys to Success in Your Exercise Program

1. *MAKE EXERCISE CONVENIENT.* Try to fit it into your lunch hour or even while you're watching TV. Just get started and remind yourself of what you hope to gain.

2. *MAKE IT FUN.* There is nothing worse than being bored or hating what you are doing. Find something you enjoy. If you like to play tennis, do that. If walking is your thing, walk every chance you get. Rollerblade with your children, hike with a friend, or get out your bike and start riding around your neighborhood.

3. *ENJOY VARIETY.* Mix it up. You don't have to walk every day! You can take a bike ride one day, walk the next, and roller blade in the park the third day.

4. *ADD MUSIC TO THE ROUTINE.* Listening to music may make exercising more enjoyable, and it often adds extra motivation to a workout. Choose your favorite tunes and see if the addition doesn't liven up your workout.

5. *EXERCISE WITH A PARTNER OR FRIEND.* As was mentioned above, a partner can provide accountability and encouragement. When you commit to someone else, you have added motivation to make the time and fulfill your commitment, but you also add fun! If you prefer a solo workout, that's fine too. Just decide what works best for you and get moving.

Warm-ups and Cooldowns[59]

It's important to warm up and cool down for at least five minutes as part of your routine. Warming up slowly increases your heart rate, getting more blood to your muscles to ready them for your workout. A cooldown allows your heart to slow down gradually. Your warm-up and cooldown don't have to be complicated. They merely involve going a little slower than usual. For example, if you're walking, start at a leisurely pace for five to six minutes and then pick up the pace by pumping your arms.

A cooldown should be built into your routine to slow down little by little. If you've been walking fast, walk slower to cool down. Stretching for a few minutes at the end of a workout is also a good idea. Research suggests that cooling down may protect your heart, relax your muscles, and keep you from getting hurt.

Incorporate Three Types of Exercise

To keep from getting into a rut, purposefully integrate different components of exercise. Variety is the secret to a solid fitness program. We recommend incorporating three components into your program:

1. ALTERNATE AEROBIC EXERCISES. Aerobic exercise burns body fat. Work your muscles differently by integrating more than one aerobic exercise into your routine. All of these aerobic activities can be alternated on any given day: walking, biking, jogging, tennis, or swimming.

For aerobic exercise, use this routine:

1. Warm up for about five minutes.
2. Slowly increase your pace until you reach your target heart zone.
3. Sustain this zone for twelve to fifteen minutes.
4. Keep moving in some way or other for ten more minutes.
5. Cool down for about five minutes.
6. Slowly decrease your pace and bring your body back to a resting level.
7. Then stretch the muscles you used for at least three minutes.

2. STRENGTH TRAINING. Strength training builds strong muscles and bones. To do this, you can exercise at home or a gym or fitness center. Hand weights or even two soup cans are fine for a beginner. Weight

training strengthens and tones muscles, and it slows bone loss and builds bone density. Other benefits include improved flexibility and mobility, more controlled blood pressure, a decrease in lower back, arthritic, and joint pain. We recommend strength training two to three days per week. Target each of the following areas of your body with strength-training exercise: arms, chest, shoulders, abs, back, buttocks, thighs, and calves.

If you are a beginner, use dumbbells rather than barbells. Begin with one hand at a time in order to get a more balanced workout. If you are strength training for fitness, do ten to twelve repetitions (reps) of each exercise for each major muscle group. If you desire to bulk up, do more sets (a set is a series of reps that are done in succession), or use heavier weights and decrease your reps. To provide variety, vary your program for strength training by using free weights one day, resistance bands another day, and machines at the gym a third day.

Always make sure you know the correct posture for the strength-training exercise and that your movements are slow and controlled. It is important to use a weight you can lift at least ten times, but no more than twelve times without tiring. If you can't do an exercise eight times in a row, your weights are too heavy. If it is easy to do the exercise twelve times in a row, your weights are too light.

3. STRETCHING. Stretching is easy to do yet has many benefits. It can improve your flexibility, blood flow, range of motion, and strength, as well as prevent your muscles from getting tight after doing other exercises. Stretching also relieves tension and stress. It's a great exercise in that you don't have to set aside a special time or place for it. Whether you're at home or at work, you can stand up, push your arms toward the ceiling, and stretch. Stretch slowly and only enough to feel tightness, not pain. If it starts to hurt, stop stretching before the stretch reflex is activated, which causes your muscles to contract instead of extending.

But you shouldn't stretch cold muscles, so do a few warm-ups first. Within your exercise routine, try to include stretching for ten minutes, at least three to five days a week. Repeat each stretch three to five times. Before you begin each exercise, exhale, then relax into the stretch. Hold the stretch for up to thirty seconds—less if you are new to stretching or start to feel uncomfortable. Here are stretches to target the various muscles of the body:

Neck

In either a standing or sitting position, ease your right ear toward your right shoulder. Gently lower your left shoulder. Slowly move your head closer to your right shoulder with your right hand. Release and then do the other side. When you are finished, shrug your shoulders, hold, and release.

Face forward. Turn your head slowly to the right and stop at the point of resistance. Hold. Gradually bring your head back to the middle. Repeat this head movement toward the left. After you have finished, lower your chin to your chest. Keep your shoulders back. Hold and release.

Shoulders

In either a standing or sitting position, extend your right arm straight across your chest. With your left hand, pull your right elbow into your chest. Hold and release. Then, switch arms and repeat.

Next, raise one arm straight up over your head. Stretch it as far as you can without bending your body. Turn the palm of your hand upward and push toward the ceiling several times. Release and repeat with your other arm. For a greater stretching movement, bend to the left at your waist as you reach with your right arm. Hold, release, and switch sides and repeat.

Triceps

In either a standing or sitting position, reach your right arm up behind your head as if to scratch the upper center of your back. (Your arm makes an inverted V by your ear.) Reach over your head with your left hand and slowly lower your right elbow. Hold and release. Switch your arms and repeat.

Biceps

With the palm of your hand up, extend your right arm out in front of you. Using your left hand, take the fingers of your right hand and pull them toward the floor. You'll want to keep your right arm straight in front of you, parallel to the floor. Switch arms and repeat.

Forearms

In a standing or sitting position, extend your right arm out in front of you, placing your palm down. With your other hand, take the fingers of your right hand and pull them slowly toward your shoulder. Hold and release. Switch arms and repeat.

Chest

Standing tall, clasp your hands behind your back. Squeeze your shoulder blades toward each other and lift your chest up and out. If you can, raise your hands and arms. It's important to keep your lower back from arching. Hold, release, and repeat.

Standing in a doorway, rest your right forearm against the doorframe. Bend your right arm in a 90-degree angle at the elbow. Slowly lean forward until you feel a comfortable stretch in your chest muscles. Hold and release. Repeat on the other side.

Back

Lie on your back with your legs extended. Clasping your right knee with your hands, slowly pull it toward your chest as far as you can without feeling discomfort. Hold. Slowly release. Switch legs and repeat. When you are finished, hug both knees to your chest. Hold and release.

Get on your hands and knees with your face and eyes looking forward. Exhale slowly while you allow your head to sag slowly toward the floor. At the same time, arch your back toward the ceiling. Hold in your stomach muscles. Hold, then release, bringing your back to the original position.

To stretch your upper back, extend your arms in front of you at shoulder height while in a standing or sitting position. Clasp your fingers together. Lower your head and turn the palms of your hands out. Round your shoulders and back, extending your arms out even farther. Hold and release.

To stretch the muscles that run alongside your back, stand up and place your feet shoulder-width apart. Link your fingers together and turn your palms upward, reaching toward the ceiling. Slowly bend to one side. Hold, and then return to the middle. Repeat on the other side.

Calves

In a standing position, extend your arms in front of you. Put your hands shoulder-width apart on a wall. Move back a couple of feet. Keeping your legs straight and your feet and heels on the floor, lean into the wall. Hold and release.

Stand on a step. Hold onto a railing or the back of a chair and allow your heels to hang off the edge of the step, lower than the position of your toes. Rise up on your toes slowly and hold for several seconds. Then, slowly lower your weight onto your heels.

Ankles

Sitting on a chair, extend your legs out in front of you with your feet one or two inches off the ground. Flex your ankles and feet toward you and hold. Then, slowly point your toes and feet downward away from you and hold. Release.

Increasing the Routine

To continue making headway in your program, eventually you will need to increase the frequency, intensity, and length of workout time. Exercising a little harder each week enables you to improve without spending more time working out. If you want to lose weight and boost your cardio-endurance, increase both the frequency and the duration of your workouts.

For the greatest overall health benefits, experts recommend twenty to thirty minutes of vigorous physical activity, such as aerobic dancing, brisk walking, or swimming three or more times a week, and some type of muscle strengthening activity, such as weight resistance or stretching at least twice a week. However, if you are unable to do this level of activity, you can improve your health by performing thirty minutes or more of moderate-intensity physical activity over the course of a day at least five times each week.[60] Such activity would include walking up stairs, walking all or part of the way to work, using a push mower to cut grass, or playing an active game with children.

Any type of physical activity you choose to do, be they vigorous activities such as running or aerobic dancing, or moderate-intensity activities such as walking or household work, will increase the number of calories your body uses. The key to successful weight control and improved overall health is to make physical activity a part of your daily life.

Research has shown that little bursts of activity throughout the day can increase your calorie burn up to a startling 500 calories or more per day.[61] These little bursts are simple and easy. Try to get up once every hour for a one- or two-minute burst of activity.

· Do standing squats as you blow-dry or curl your hair.

· Pace or march in place while you talk on the phone.

· Take the stairs whenever possible.

· Squeeze your buttock muscles and zip up your abs as you stand in line at the grocery store or while manning the fax machine.

Seven Outdoor Cardio Workouts that Burn Fat Fast

If you'd like to step up your workout and burn more calories, try these seven ideas for a cardio workout:

1. BICYCLING

Calorie burn per fifteen minutes:
Road biking, 136; trail or mountain biking, 145

Did you like to ride a bicycle as a kid? If so, you may want to try road or trail cycling. Cycling is a great no-impact to low-impact activity to help burn calories. Do it long enough and intensely enough in order to keep your heart rate in the fat-burning zone. For rougher terrain, you may want to try a mountain bike. These bikes have wider tires and are heavy. You can also buy a larger seat for your bike to avoid becoming sore. Make sure the bike you buy has a weight rating at least as high as your own weight.

Bicycling enables you to get outdoors and explore your neighborhood and area parks. It's also a great way to get around when you're on vacation. Many cities feature bicycle trails that protect cyclists from traffic. And mountain or trail riding is a great activity to get in touch with nature, but do stay on trails for your safety.

Whether you take to the road or the trail is your decision. Riding on roads will give you a more predictable, steady workout with fewer bumps and unexpected turns, but you will have to deal with traffic. Trail riding offers the potential for a greater workout for your upper body as you maneuver through uneven terrain and bumps.

Be cautious your first time out: Be sure you know where you are located so that you can make it back. Use good form to avoid stiffness. When cycling, regularly arch and round your back as you ride. When gripping the handlebar, keep your elbows unlocked. Keeping a loose grip will also keep you from having tingling hands.

2. Cardio Kickboxing

Calorie burn per fifteen minutes: 170

Do you want a fun way to relieve fat-generating stress while getting a great workout that burns those calories and tones your major muscles at the same time? Cardio kickboxing provides a positive format to help you release tension and aggression. Because it's not about kicking higher or punching harder than everyone else, it can easily be modified to suit your needs. The old adage of "no pain, no gain" simply does not apply to this form of exercise. You will finish sessions feeling better both mentally and physically.

Give your body a chance to get used to the movements, even if you're a seasoned exerciser. "Keep your kicks low and don't punch with a lot of intensity," says one instructor certified by the American Council on Exercise. "Listen to your body. If you are tired, take a break. If you get thirsty, drink some water. If you feel discomfort, stop. It's important to pace yourself, but do challenge yourself during the workout."

If you leave class early, remember to cool down and stretch on your own. Kickboxing classes provide a warm-up with a stretch as well as twenty to forty minutes of cardio work that includes kicking and punching drills. Some classes will also have running and skipping, which can be modified by marching in place. Music is a driving force in many cardio kickboxing workouts. Some instructors may be open to you suggesting songs or certain styles of music. The variety within this form of exercise, as well as personal enjoyment, will help you stay with your program.

3. DANCING

Calorie burn per fifteen minutes: Jitterbug and tap, 80; country and western, disco, Irish step, line, swing, and flamenco, 75; cha-cha, 50

Do you love to dance the night away? You'll be pleasantly surprised to learn that you burn fifty or more calories for every fifteen minutes you do the cha-cha or the bump. Some forms of dancing burn more calories than others. Slower dances like waltzes can burn up to fifty calories while jazz dancing can burn more than eighty calories for the same fifteen-minute span.

If you're worried about not being able to keep up with the rest of your dance class, feel free to stand back and watch. One dance instructor comments, "Standing behind someone who seems to know what they're doing is a great trick. In a dance class, you're very dependent on the people who are a little more advanced than you."

Before you begin to dance, breathe deeply and shrug off the worries of the day. Mastering the moves will enable you to begin to improvise, create your own movements, and be more expressive. With dance, there are no limits! Choose from any number of ethnic styles or traditional forms to find a form that's right for you.

4. HIKING

Calorie burn per fifteen minutes: 120

You can soothe your soul and burn those calories at the same time by hitting the trail. There's nothing like being surrounded by trees and chirping birds to help you forget that you're burning calories as you walk. If you are a beginner, try a well-traveled, level trail. Have the right footwear, hat, and sunscreen handy. And, don't forget to stretch when you finish.

Turn your hike into a special occasion by bringing along a picnic lunch. Relax and enjoy the scenery. There are endless trails which allow you to hike up mountains, along rivers, and even through city parks. Give yourself permission to go at a slower pace if necessary, because you are exercising and whether you walk a little slower for a period of time is irrelevant—what's important is the fact that you are outside and moving around!

5. IN-LINE SKATING

Calorie burn per fifteen minutes: 84–119, depending on intensity

Zoom off the calories! Tone your troubled spots! You can cover a lot of ground fast with in-line skating. However, just learning how to use the skates is good exercise. It takes a lot of energy to do it correctly when you are a beginner. Take a little extra time and be sure you know how to use the heel brakes on the skates. If you are just starting out, find an empty parking lot with a smooth, level surface. Your neighborhood roads can be quite bumpy, which may cause your shins to hurt. Master the basics and then try a squatting position, or use long, graceful strides, which will make in-line skating feel more like ice-skating than roller-skating. Try going uphill for an even greater burn and overall workout.

6. SWIMMING LAPS

Calorie burn per fifteen minutes: 136

Swimming laps is the best choice for a total-body workout and stress reducer. Unlike other activities, water workouts exercise both the upper and lower body. And because of the buoyancy of the water, water exercise doesn't stress your joints the way other activities do. You can bend and move your body in water in ways you can't on land. Swimming is an ideal exercise if you're overweight or recovering from an injury.

To find a pool near you, check out your local YMCA or community center. Also, if you don't want to fight for lane space during your first few sessions, ask when the pool is least crowded. Don't be discouraged if you can do only one or two laps at first. Swim as long as you comfortably can, rest for a few minutes, and then start swimming again. In time, you'll be able to swim farther and longer. Because doing the same stroke lap after lap can get boring, try the breaststroke, freestyle, backstroke, and even the sidestroke for variety and an enjoyable swimming workout.

If you never learned to swim, you should know that it isn't necessary to know how to swim in order to work out in water. You can do shallow-water exercises without swimming. Just make sure the water level is between your waist and your chest. If the water is too shallow, it will be hard to move your arms underwater. If the water is too deep, it will be hard to keep your feet touching the pool bottom.

7. STEP AEROBICS

Calorie burn per fifteen minutes: 102, depending on your weight

Strengthen and tone your leg and bun muscles while burning calories with step aerobics. You step on and off a platform about two or three feet long that rests on the floor or atop one or more risers. Once you learn the basic moves—getting on and off the platform, over, and across it, you are ready for routines led by an instructor. If you're a beginner, start with a platform height of four to six inches. If your knees are bent more than 90 degrees, your step is too high.

Focus on the arm movements after you have the steps down. Keep your neck and back straight, shoulders back, pelvis tucked, abdominal muscles pulled in, and chest lifted. Lean from your ankles when stepping onto the platform. The music and the group interaction provide extra stimulus for sticking with this form of exercise.

Try Walking

If the above seven options sound a bit too strenuous, there is always walking. Walking is a great form of exercise and something most people can do. Do light stretching before and after you walk, and warm up with five minutes of slow walking. Increase your speed for the next five or more minutes. Then, cool down by walking slowly for the last five minutes. Make sure you stand up straight, lift your rib cage, and look straight ahead (but keep your shoulders relaxed). This will let your spine curve in a natural, healthy position. Swing your arms and move at a steady pace. This will also help keep your fingers from swelling.

Walking should be enjoyable. Try walking with a friend or pet, and walk in places you enjoy, like a park or shopping mall. Your walking partner(s) should be able to walk with you on the same schedule and at the same speed. If possible, walk at least three times per week, and add two to three minutes per week to the fast walk. If you walk less than three times per week, increase the fast walk segment more slowly. Over time, make it a goal to walk faster, farther, and for longer periods of time. The more you walk, the better you will feel, and the more calories you will burn.

When you walk, always think about safety. Walk in the daytime or at night in well-lit areas. We recommend walking with another person or in a group, especially at night. You can even notify your local police station of your group's walking time and route, if you desire. Become aware of your surroundings and leave headphones off. And, leave your jewelry at home![63]

A Common Problem for Walkers—Heel Pain

It's an annoying reality that all walkers face one day. The older you get, the more likely you are to experience the stabbing heel pain known as plantar fasciitis. *That's because, as you grow older, the ligaments in your foot stretch and lose some of their supportive quality. Your foot can then over-pronate (lean inward) more easily, stretching tissues on the sole of your foot beyond their normal length. Over time, this tissue (called plantar fascia) becomes inflamed and sometimes even tears, causing pain.*[62]

Taking anti-inflammatory medication or simply waiting for the pain to sub-side on its own won't solve the problem and could, in fact, lead to a more serious injury that may take months to heal. Here are four steps you can take now to stop the throbbing.

1. REPLACE YOUR WALKING SHOES BEFORE THEY WEAR OUT. Buy shoes at least every 300 miles (or four or five months) if you walk around fifteen miles per week.

2. BE SURE TO STRETCH. Tight calf muscles create additional pres-sure on the tissues under the foot. Get in the habit of stretching regularly before and after your walks. Start by standing about eighteen inches from a wall with your palms on the wall. Extend your right leg back about two feet, and bend your left knee. Keep your right leg straight, pressing your right heel into the ground. Your toes should be pointing forward. Hold for fifteen seconds, and then switch legs. If you experience heel soreness, stretch ten times with each leg, twice a day.

3. CURB YOUR WALKS. If supportive shoes or inserts ease your dis-comfort (ask for help at your local sports store), then it's fine to continue walking. Just avoid hills or roads that are sloped toward the shoulder. But if your pain is severe, you may have to take time off. Check with your doctor to see if cycling, swimming, or another activity might be a good sub-stitute for your walks.

4. SEE A PODIATRIST OR ORTHOPEDIC SPECIALIST. If you don't notice any improvement within one or two weeks, you should see a doctor.

For some of you, exercise will be your biggest challenge. When you are overweight, exercise is difficult because it physically hurts the body to move all that weight around. Part of the work will be finding movement that isn't painful—like water aerobics, or exercises that don't put pressure on the joints.

We know it's embarrassing to go to a public pool to do aquatic exercise. Putting on a bathing suit in public is not for the fainthearted. Several years ago however, something terrific happened in my community that gave me (Dr. Linda) renewed hope regarding this issue. As I pulled together a multidisciplinary team of health care providers to work with my obese clients, I listened to the pain, embarrassment, and shame they faced when they tried to exercise. The exercise physiologist on our team responded with a wonderful plan.

We negotiated with a local YMCA for a private room to lead exercise classes. These classes would not be open to the public—only to my clients, but at a much reduced fee. The instructor led the classes in a way that minimized their physical pain yet slowly but steadily got the group moving. In the privacy of that room, organized exercise was finally a fun option. We also set up private hours for use of the swimming pool. In the water, movement was so much easier on their bodies.

I can't tell you how grateful these clients were for the opportunity to exercise without feeling humiliated. They cried, we cried, and the weight began to drop off. Because a few people cared enough to be empathetic and support people with a particular need, these hurting people found healing.

Every one of those clients wanted to make changes, but embarrassment had kept them from trying. Please don't allow negative past experiences to stop you from doing what is in your heart to do. You can be victorious in this journey. God knows your physical and emotional pain and isn't judging you, and there are people who can and will support you in this endeavor.

As you begin to exercise, you may encounter people who don't understand and who may judge you. Yet God sees and knows what you are going through. As Paul admonishes us in Philippians 3:13-14, " . . . forgetting those things which are behind and reaching forward to those things which are ahead, [we] press toward the goal" (NKJV, emphasis added). Don't focus on what you can't do or how others may perceive you. Instead, reflect on each small step you make and recognize those steps for what they are—individual acts of courage.

Exercise isn't an option if you want to reap the benefits of a healthy life. Whatever your pleasure, there is an activity that is right for you, but it's up to you to find that exercise and to get moving. Whether it's walking, aerobics, weight lifting, stretching, or even taking the stairs instead of the elevator, each small change will make a difference in your health, weight maintenance, and mental health. So get motivated and get moving so you can lose it for life!

7

— Coming Out (of the Eating Closet) —

November 21, 2003—What a week! Hands down, this has been one of the toughest weeks I've faced since embarking on this healthy lifestyle journey. Needless to say, my emotions have been all over the place. In the past, I have always stuffed away the sad or emotional times by eating large amounts of comfort food until I was emotionally numb, i.e., safe. I have now stopped medicating with food, and it's incredible to actually "feel" my emotions—good and bad. Of course, some days I want to run to the refrigerator and comfort myself with food. But, amazing as it sounds, this is when I'm learning to press into God even harder and ask Him to walk me through the emotions at hand. I can't share all I've gone through this week, but I can say it's a miracle I have not gone back to my old ways. It's confirmation to me that the Lord has begun a good work in my life. I am now down 92 pounds. I have 8 pounds to go until I reach the halfway mark. Praise God.

December 17, 2003—Imagine living your life numb. Never really experiencing true happiness, joy, sadness, etc. In this state, life just sort of passes you by while you exist. Sadly enough, this is how I have lived most of my life. I've learned that this was how I protected myself from past hurts, humiliations, letdowns, and unforgiveness [sic] in my life. The good news is that with the Lord's constant guiding in this journey, I have made a U-turn. Let me tell you, it is an incredible thing to feel, to really live life experiencing the good and the not-so-good times. It is so much better than simply existing in a numb state, day after day after day.

I have also realized that not only did I not want to feel, but I was uncomfortable when my kids felt too. I have always said things like "stop crying," or "you're okay, it's not that bad," when my kids were hurting. I thought I was protecting them, but I now realize that I should have allowed them to feel their emotions. It's healthy to have good days and bad days. It's healthy to let them cry it out when they hurt, to scream out when excited, and to voice their fears when afraid. From now on, I am asking the Lord to help my kids and me learn to face our emotions and walk through them head on, so we can continue to grow and become the people God created us to be.

—CATHY

Cathy has come out of the eating closet! For the first time in a long time, she is beginning to feel emotions she used to numb out with food. And sometimes she feels overwhelmed, like a dam is breaking and she'll be swept away by the force of her emotions. But we love Cathy's new response—to press into God even harder and know He will walk her through the emotions she feels. God is faithful and can be trusted. He may not always remove Cathy from difficulty, but He promises His comfort, peace, and presence no matter what.

What is so encouraging about this brave sister in the Lord is that she is not asking God to remove her feelings or the feelings of her children. Cathy is beyond "the quick fix, instant solution" God concept that typifies the spiritual move many people make. Instead, she is asking God to help her and her kids face the feelings and allow the experience to produce growth. This truly is how we can continue to grow and become the people God created us to be. There is no lifestyle, no matter how healthy, that will free you from negative emotions or horrible pain. But you can find a way to face those moments, resolve them, and grow from the experience, if you allow God to help you.

The Gift of Emotional Pain

One of our favorite physicians is Dr. Paul Brand, a man who dedicated his life to helping people with leprosy. What struck him while working with these patients was their inability to feel pain—literally, the patients would become injured and not know it! Because pain is an important warning signal that something is wrong, Dr. Brand spent his life trying to find a way to give his patients the "gift of pain."

Physical pain is necessary to our functioning. It is part of God's design for our bodies because it signals there is a problem to which we should attend. Emotional pain is similar. It signals there is a problem God wants to heal. Cathy is learning this for the first time in her life. Rather than protect herself from emotional pain by using food as her numbing agent, she is taking courageous steps to walk through past hurts and problems. When we see emotional pain as the symptom that leads us to depend on God and turn to Him for healing, we begin to understand its purpose.

Granted, you may be thinking, *If emotional pain is a gift, please don't give it to me!* But think about the times in your life when you have grown the most. Were they during the mountaintop experiences or in the lows of the valleys? Most of us grow during valley experiences, those difficult times in our lives when we can turn one of two ways—toward a more intimate relationship with God or away from Him. And when we choose to go to God, we grow and mature.

Cathy is leaving a legacy for her children. She is breaking a family pattern and teaching her children to feel emotional pain and deal with it. What a gift to give the next generation! As this family learns to feel the good and the bad, they will realize they can tolerate much more than they ever thought possible. No longer will they have to hide from emotional feelings, because they have found freedom!

Are You an Emotional Eater?

Cathy admits she is an emotional eater. She anesthetizes herself with food so she doesn't have to feel negative emotions. Like so many overeaters, this woman was unaware that emotions were at the root of her hunger. Perhaps you are like Cathy and haven't made the connection between overeating and emotions. If not, now is the time to take a deeper look at your relationship with food. The twenty questions below will help you decide if you are an emotional eater.

1. Do I think about food often or all the time?
2. Do I eat to relieve tension, worry, or upsets?
3. Do I eat when I am bored?
4. Do I continue to eat after I feel full, sometimes to the point of feeling sick?
5. Does eating relieve my anxiety?
6. Do I eat without thinking?
7. Do I have to clean my plate?
8. Do I eat in secret or hide food?
9. Do I eat quickly, shoving in the food?
10. Do I feel guilty after I eat?
11. Do I eat small portions in front of people, but go back for more food when people aren't around?
12. Do I binge (eat large amounts of food in a short time)?

13. Can I eat one serving, or do I eat the entire amount (a bag of cookies, or the whole half gallon of ice cream)?
14. Do I feel out of control and impulsive when eating?
15. Do I eat when I am not physically hungry?
16. Do I lie to myself about how much I really eat?
17. Do I have trouble tolerating negative feelings?
18. Do I have impulse problems in other areas of my life (shopping, gambling, sex, alcohol, pornography, drugs)?
19. Have I been on numerous diets over the years?
20. Do I experience constant weight fluctuations?

If you answered yes to all of these, well, you are probably so depressed you are eating right now, or you are crying so hard you cannot read on. If you answered yes to several of these questions, chances are you are an emotional eater. This means that feelings often trigger your desire to eat. This is not an easy topic, but it is imperative to get to the root of why you are eating. In fact, it is the key to unlocking your weight problem—*when you stop eating depends on why you are eating.*

Emotional eating can be learned early as a child. Food can be used to comfort, or it can become a trusted friend. Children often use food in response to physical or sexual abuse, or growing up in the home of an alcoholic or mentally ill parent, or in response to any number of difficult circumstances. When boundaries are violated, as in cases of abuse, or nurturing is unstable or unpredictable, as in cases of neglect and addiction, or loss is experienced in significant ways, as in situations involving divorce or death, children often turn to food for comfort. Eating calms the anxiety, numbs out trauma and abuse, and soothes the troubled soul.

Other people become emotional eaters as a result of trauma or stress experienced later in life. The trigger might be an unhealthy relationship, death, illness, or a job loss. In my own case, I (Dr. Linda) used food to cope with my brother's death. He was killed when the airplane he was on exploded over New Delhi, India. (We now believe the plane was the target of a terrorist bomb.) It happened the summer before I left for college. Between the trauma of his death and beginning my freshman year of college out of state, the losses were great. I unconsciously used food to soothe myself from all the stress and emotional pain I carried, and I gained thirty pounds before realizing eating was my new coping mechanism.

I remember feeling unprotected when my brother was killed. We were a Christian family! Where was God when that plane went down? The enemy, during a time of incredible hurt and loss, implants doubt about who God is and how He loves and cares for us. Like Eve, I listened to that gnawing, twisted voice. I made a vow to never be dependent on a man, and I wouldn't allow that kind of hurt to happen again. I would take control of my life. God could come along for the ride, but He had to take the back seat, because in my mind, He was no longer trustworthy.

Even though I grieved my brother's death, those unspoken vows caused marital problems in the early years of my marriage. What I didn't realize was how captive I was to fear. Freedom came when I renounced those old vows and then challenged the lie of my unbelief. In prayer, I asked Jesus to speak His truth to me.

As I waited before the Lord in prayer, I heard Him tell me that my life was in His hands. There is not a day I live that He hasn't numbered; in fact, my life had been in His control all along. I had to trust Him, despite my lack of understanding. I didn't have to understand my brother's death, but I did have to trust that "all things work together for good to those who love God" (Romans 8:28 NKJV). My faith was on trial, and my unbelief and doubt were choking the spiritual intimacy I desperately needed.

What Is the Answer?

Our lives, our eating, and our emotions all have spiritual ramifications. You can rely on God. God won't protect you from horrible situations or difficult emotions, but He does sustain and protect His children from hopelessness. God knows what you need, always. And through the pain and struggle of this journey, He will deliver you, if you are willing.

One of the biggest barriers to moving forward in the things God has for us is getting stuck in our emotional pain and allowing it to move us away from God. When we experience trials or suffering, we might not loudly reject God, but we may very well begin to doubt who He is and whether He truly loves and cares for us. We all have experienced hurts and disappointments in our lives. For some of us, we've had deep traumas or abuse. For others, we've experienced lost dreams, disappointments, heartaches, and relationship problems. Certainly, there is no shortage of emotional pain. And unfortunately, all that suffering can lead us down the road to anxiety, depression, and eating problems.

The reality is that putting your trust in anything or anyone but God will block your intimacy with Him. Our earthly supports, whether people or merchandise, gradually disappoint or fade away. We live in uncertain times. God wants you to look to Him first for security. He came to bring peace and comfort to those who mourn.

> He has the power to heal the brokenhearted,
> to proclaim liberty to the captive,
> to open the prison doors to those who are bound,
> to give beauty to ashes,
> and the garment of praise for the spirit of heaviness,
> that we might be called trees of righteousness,
> the planting of the Lord, that *He might be glorified.*
> (adapted from Isaiah 61:1-3, emphasis added)

Let your emotional pain lead you to Him. Become His tree planted with deep roots, trusting Him, knowing Him, so that He can transform your pain for His glory. God wants us to come to Him no matter what—so don't allow your losses and pain to turn you away from Him. The answers are found in Him. "For in Him we live and move and have our being" (Acts 17:28 NKJV).

Your loss might be the work of the enemy and something God allowed to happen. But just look at the story of Job. Job was righteous in God's eyes. He was faithful and yet lost everything because God allowed it. Job's story illustrates how we can obey God and be right in the center of His will and yet still experience great loss. And when this happens, it is very hard to understand, and harder still to accept.

Turning to food is but one choice for covering up emotional pain. But once emotional eating becomes habitual, you have to break the connection between emotions and food to get back on track. Those emotions need to be revisited, felt intensely, grieved, and released. If you struggle with emotional pain and are using food to cover up the hurt, pour out your heart to the Lord as Hannah did in 1 Samuel 1. And remember that Christ has taken your grief and carried your sorrow (Isaiah 53). He identifies with what you are going through. He intimately knows every tear you cry, and He can handle your intense feelings.

In addition to pouring your heart out to God, find someone who will listen and can be trusted with your pain. This may be a good friend, a counselor, a family member, or your spouse. The Bible instructs us to "bear one another's burdens" (Galatians 6:2 NKJV) and to intercede in prayer on behalf of others. Allow trusted people in your life to be a part of your healing journey. Often they have words of encouragement or scriptures that will uplift you and offer hope when you are feeling down.

RISE Above Emotional Eating

As you already know, physical hunger is rarely the trigger for overeating. Overeating can be stimulated by seeing food, thinking certain thoughts, learning behavior patterns, and feeling certain emotions. What we must learn is to:

1. identify the emotions associated with the urge to overeat;
2. feel those emotions and manage them, instead of allowing them to manage us;
3. work through emotional pain, grieve it, and allow God to transform it.

We can assure you that people who learn to respond to emotional difficulties without using food to numb or escape feelings have a better and longer weight loss maintenance record than those who only deal with eating and exercise. Both research and clinical experience support this reality. This is a difficult road to take, because a learned way of coping needs to be unlearned. You may feel flooded with emotions that you haven't felt in a long time, thanks to eating covering them up, but the rewards are well worth the effort.

To RISE above the challenge, here's what to expect:

REDUCE: stress where and when you can; also eating in response to negative feelings and stress.

INCREASE: confession, your ability to tolerate negative feelings, confrontation of tough issues, and assertiveness.

SUBSTITUTE: new ways to deal with emotions for eating, such as grieving for overeating.

ELIMINATE: fear, feelings of rejection and shame, and hopelessness.

Identify the Feelings

When you have the urge to eat, try to identify what you feel. This sounds easy enough, but if you have been taught to ignore feelings, particularly negative emotions like anger, envy, or pride, it may be more difficult. Negative emotions are part of our human condition and must be dealt with in a healthy and biblical way. Emotions aren't wrong or bad, but what you do with an emotion counts.

I (Steve) heard a comedian do a comedy routine around the fact that there are about 2,000 emotions and men are only able to feel between three or four, or only know what three or four are! I hope it is not that bad for us men. It is so important that we learn to identify what feelings we are experiencing.

After my divorce I began to feel deep emotional pain like I had never experienced before. I hurt at the core of who I was. I did not try to eat or drink it away. The pain was too intense and destroyed my desire for anything. I cried and sometimes wailed in my despair. Initially, I told myself all I was feeling was a generic pain that all experience. It wasn't until just a few months ago that I really got in touch with what that pain really was: pure fear to the degree I would even label it terror. I was afraid of what would happen to my daughter. I was afraid of what would happen to my ministry. I was afraid of everything that could go wrong as a result of the divorce. My faith was at an all-time low while my fear raged on. And because I did not identify the fear as the source of my pain, I didn't deal with it in the counseling I was involved with. As a result, that fear stayed with me for far too long. It was only when I acknowledged it and addressed my lack of faith that the fear subsided and my pain had a purpose.

I hope you come to identify the feelings you have and then start to deal with them openly and honestly so they will no longer control any part of your life. The end result will be that you are no longer an emotional eater compelled to eat in a futile effort to medicate the emptiness within your soul.

Anger

This is the most reported emotion tied to overeating. People eat when they are angry! Anger feels uncomfortable and is often confused with a need to eat. It's interesting to note that women, more so than men, have trouble acknowledging anger. This may have to do with parent training (nice girls don't get mad), corporate game playing rules (just look pretty and don't say anything), or other societal messages women receive.

Though it is sometimes viewed as bad, anger is a biblical reality. Cain was so angry, he murdered his brother (Genesis 4:5-8); Simeon and Levi took revenge for their sister's rape (Genesis 49:5-7); Herod was angry toward the wise men for deceiving him (Matthew 2:16); the people of Nazareth were angry with Jesus (Luke 4:28); and Paul felt anger toward Ananias (Acts 23:1-3). The list goes on and on. Keep in mind that when Jesus took the form of man, He experienced every emotion, including anger.

The biblical directive given in Ephesians 4:26 (NASB) is, "Be angry, and yet do not sin." This scripture affirms anger as part of our human nature but also tells us not to sin in response to that emotion. Yet anger will not go away on its own. To be rid of it requires recognizing anger, acknowledging you have it, and then dealing with it according to these biblical guidelines:

JAMES 1:19—Be quick to listen, slow to speak and slow to become angry.

PROVERBS 29:11—A fool gives full vent to his anger, but a wise man keeps himself under control.

PROVERBS 15:1—A gentle answer turns away wrath, but a harsh word stirs up anger.

MATTHEW 6:14—"For if you forgive men when they sin against you, your heavenly Father will also forgive you."

PSALM 4:4—In your anger do not sin; when you are on your beds, search your hearts and be silent.

1 PETER 5:7—Cast all your anxiety on him because he cares for you.

PROVERBS 22:24—Don't hang out with angry people; don't keep company with hotheads. (MSG)

Fatigue

Many of us overeat when we are tired. Food is often used to energize us. If you are a workaholic, you've probably used food to keep your energy level up. Or maybe you use food to ease tension from being overly tired. If you've had a horrendous day at the office, overdone it by drinking too much coffee and snacking on chocolate for quick recharging, you may crave carbohydrates at night to calm you down. Overeating happens more often when we are tired and our defenses are down. We take a careless attitude and dive into snacking.

If you are tired, rest is what you need. Food may give you a temporary surge, but you will end up feeling more sluggish and still tired in the long run. Rest, exercise, and eat well. Eating when you are tired only compounds your problems. Rest is biblical—even God rested after creating the world.

PSALM 37:7—Rest in the LORD and wait patiently for Him. (NKJV)

MATTHEW 11:28-30—"Are you tired? Worn out? Burned out on religion? Come to me. Get away with me and you'll recover your life. I'll show you how to take a real rest. Walk with me and work with me—watch how I do it. Learn the unforced rhythms of grace. I won't lay anything heavy or ill-fitting on you. Keep company with me and you'll learn to live freely and lightly." (MSG)

HEBREWS 4:1—For as long, then, as that promise of resting in him pulls us on to God's goal for us, we need to be careful that we're not disqualified. (MSG)

HEBREWS 4:9—The promise of "arrival" and "rest" is still there for God's people. (MSG)

Depression

When you feel down, it's easy to try and eat those feelings away. People who eat when they feel depressed usually go for dairy products like ice cream or cheese—and of course, chocolate! These foods tend to provide a boost by giving the brain a neurochemical lift. But eating doesn't take away depression; it only masks it.

Your most powerful weapon against depression is praise. We are told in Isaiah 61:3 to put on a garment of praise for a spirit of despair. Don't wait to feel like you want to praise. Do it no matter what you feel like. Praise God for who He is. Praise is the anecdote to feeling down. Let His praise be in your mouth continuously (Psalm 34:1), and the Lord will lift your spirit.

If you struggle with clinical depression, there is nothing wrong with going on an antidepressant to help stabilize your mood and correct brain chemistry. Taking medication does not demonstrate a lack of faith. Antidepressants are simply agents used to get you living well again by restoring proper brain functioning. All healing comes through God, but He does use miracles and medicine to accomplish His purposes. You may need to see a doctor and/or a therapist to help with depression.

Loneliness

When you are lonely, you may overeat instead of engaging in activities that could end your loneliness. Food can become a trusted friend who is always with you and always available. Therefore, you must find other ways to deal with loneliness. Join an organization, volunteer your time, enroll in a class, become active with a charity, attend a church function, or make the first move and call someone you'd like to befriend.

The Duchess of York, Sarah Ferguson, lost her mother to a divorce when she was twelve years old. Her mother left her and her father to marry another man and move to Argentina. Since that time, Sarah describes herself as an emotional eater. "I overate to compensate for my feelings. I didn't want to express to my mother that I was angry or sad that she'd left me."[64] She admits that she was blind to the emotional triggers that set off her eating as an adult. Loneliness can be that trigger.

Inadequacy

When you don't feel good about yourself, you can eat to cover up feelings of inadequacy. Most people wrestle with self-doubt from time to time, but if you have a constant feeling of being inadequate, you may be tying your eating to that feeling. We are all inadequate because we are human. You must learn to accept your weaknesses and flaws and not dwell on them. And when you feel inadequate or weak, it helps to know that God is strong and can work through you anyway.

Make a list of your strengths and weaknesses. Try to focus on those things you do well. Then ask God to help you with your weaknesses. By His Spirit, He is able to accomplish much, even with your limitations (Zechariah 4:6). Turning to food will not help you accomplish anything. In fact, it leads to more feelings of inadequacy because of weight gain.

This is an area that has plagued me (Steve) since I was a child. My first problem was an obsession with others and comparing myself to them, trying to figure out where I was on the food chain. I wanted so much and to do so much while always feeling I had too little. It wasn't until I finally realized that the curse of not being as talented or having as much as others was actually a gift.

The gift was knowing that God had done things through me in spite of my inadequacies rather than because of my strengths. It was a gift to see that although I did not measure up, God used me to become part of His kingdom building project. If you start to look at your emotions and find that inadequacy is at the top of the list, give up on trying to feel better about yourself and start focusing on feeling better about God. Look at what God has done through you. Look at what God has allowed to happen in your life even though you did not have it all together or have all that others had.

Insecurity

If you eat because you feel insecure, no amount of food will change that feeling. The only place you are truly secure is in your relationship with God. A multitude of scriptures speak to who we are in Christ—we are loved, forgiven, saved by grace through faith, joint heirs with Christ, blessed with all spiritual blessings, sons and daughters of God, complete in Him, and so much more. It may help you to do a study on scriptures related to our security in Christ. Here are a few to get you started:

PSALM 34:4—I sought the LORD, and he answered me; he delivered me from all my fears.

DEUTERONOMY 31:8—"The LORD himself goes before you and will be with you; he will never leave you nor forsake you. Do not be afraid; do not be discouraged."

ROMANS 8:28—And we know that in all things God works for the good of those who love him, who have been called according to his purpose.

2 CORINTHIANS 1:21-22—Now it is God who makes both us and you stand firm in Christ. He anointed us, set his seal of ownership on us, and put his Spirit in our hearts as a deposit, guaranteeing what is to come.

Guilt

Guilt is only healthy when it relates to sin. We should feel guilty when we go against God's Word and sin. But once we confess that sin, it is gone and forgotten. To hang on to guilt serves no good purpose and can be cause for overeating. Jesus does not accuse (John 5:45) nor condemn you (Romans 8:1). When you own your mistakes and take responsibility, you must let go of condemnation and unhealthy guilt—to not do so is to ignore the power of the blood covenant over past sins. You may intellectually know that Jesus died on the cross to take your sins, yet be unable to get past your mistakes. So you walk around carrying tremendous guilt and shame, yet Christ died so you could give Him these sins and burdens. Hand them over and walk with your head held high.

In 2 Corinthians 7:9-10 we see what God is really after when we do something wrong:

Now I [Paul] am happy, not because you were made sorry, but because your sorrow led you to repentance. For you became sorrowful as God intended. . . . Godly sorrow brings repentance that leads to salvation and leaves no regret, but worldly sorrow brings death.

Godly sorrow moves us to change. It motivates us toward God and relationship with Him. So feel the guilt, confess it, and then turn it into a spiritual experience of godly sorrow that increases your character.

Shame

Shame takes you nowhere but the refrigerator. Shame comes when you've done something improper or wrong and you internalize "badness" because of it. Shame says, "I *am* a mistake," not "I *made* a mistake." Shame often develops from a message that you are bad, weak, or unloved. Parents, teachers, friends, boyfriends, spouses, and co-workers can humiliate, belittle, and criticize rather than deal with inappropriate behavior a better way. If you struggle with shame from overeating, you aren't alone. Read this journal entry:

> *A few years ago I went with a group of friends to a theme park. We waited in line for almost an hour to ride their largest roller coaster, and our excitement level was huge by the time we actually took our seats on the ride. I'll never forget what happened next.*
>
> *Each car held four people. For some reason the car I was in was having a problem with the safety bar locking. The ride operator came by to assist us. He pushed the bar down, attempting to safely lock us in. As he did this, I felt extreme pain as the bar pinched an area of my outer thigh against the metal seat. He didn't realize it was my large legs causing the problem, so he continued to jiggle and*

pushed down on the bar a few more times with all his strength. The pain was excruciating, and I could feel the blood running down my leg, but I was frozen with shame and unable to speak.

The young ride operator finally realized what the problem was and, in front of everyone, said, "I'm sorry, you're too big for this ride." I was crushed. I climbed out of the ride embarrassed and ashamed, trying not to limp, and acted like it was no big deal. Some people were laughing and snickering and others looked mortified. I started laughing and pretended not to care about what had just happened. I told my friends to go without me and, once the roller coaster was out of sight, I slipped away and cried alone. As you can imagine, I have not felt very comfortable going on carnival rides since.

—CATHY

Experiencing this kind of insensitivity can leave scars. We want you to be free of the hurt right now and not have to wait to be thinner! If you've read this entry and are feeling shame right now, here's what we want you to do. Embrace that shame and allow yourself to feel it. Understand, it's going to feel awful, but don't push it away or try to avoid it. Then ask the Lord to show you the source of that pain—a cruel word, a disappointing look, a moment of rejection. Let your mind go wherever the Holy Spirit takes you.

With that memory in mind, try to think *why* you feel shame. What thought comes to your mind? Is it *I am a bad person* or *I don't deserve to be treated nicely?* Be honest with what you are thinking. The thought is most likely a lie. Once you've identified the lie, ask Jesus to speak His truth to you. Wait and allow Him to speak truth. What do you see or hear Him say? His truth will set you free from that shame. Then, forgive the person who did or said something that created that feeling of shame.

Shame is a deep internal response of feeling unworthy in another person's eyes. It can be experienced through unkind words and actions. But understand something important. Jesus does not shame you. He sees you as worthy and valuable! He does not judge you by your weight. When He sees the shame you experience, He urges you to bring it to the cross. He died for it.

The life lived with God is a great adventure, much like the roller coaster ride. It is filled with ups and downs to be experienced. When you experience the downside, find your worth in Him and hand over the shame. He's with you on this journey and won't ask you to step out of the car. Instead, He'll ride alongside, whether you fit in the car or not. And He's whispering in your ear, "Enjoy the ride. Shame is not on you! I took it to the cross!"

Many women with lifelong weight problems were molested at a young age. They felt the shame of that molestation for years and fed the pain with food. They medicated the horror with carbohydrates and anything that would give them some sense of comfort. Essentially they took the shame of another and put it onto themselves. Though innocent, they lived out a sentence of shame that the guilty should have experienced. If this is your story, please release your shame to God. Give it up, let it go, and experience the love and acceptance that God has for you now and has always had for you.

Jealousy

People eat out of jealousy when they compare themselves to others and look only at the appearance of others. To assume because others are thin that they are happy and living a good life is to be deceived. Jesus tells us to "Stop judging by mere *appearances,* and make a right judgment" (John 7:24, emphasis added). He is not impressed with people who *seem* to be important. And Paul, in Galatians 2:6, follows Christ by saying, "As for those who seemed to be important—whatever they were makes no difference to me; God does not judge by external appearance—those men added nothing to my message." So stop comparing yourself to others. Jealousy is a very unproductive emotion.

Happiness

When things are going well, some people turn to food in order to fill up on those happy emotions. Happiness is something to be gobbled up before it disappears. Others feel they don't deserve to be happy and eat to sabotage happy feelings. We frequently see this when people are beginning to be successful with weight loss.

It's wonderful to be happy, but those feelings come and go and can't be relied upon as a gauge for eating. So when you are happy, celebrate in other ways like calling a friend, getting a massage, buying fresh flowers, or enjoying the stars on a clear night. And recognize that while happiness comes and goes, you always have joy in the Lord; joy is your strength.

PSALM 19:8—The precepts of the LORD are right, giving joy to the heart. The commands of the LORD are radiant, giving light to the eyes.

JAMES 5:13—Is any one of you in trouble? He should pray. Is anyone happy? Let him sing songs of praise.

ACTS 14:17—He has shown kindness by giving you rain from heaven and crops in their seasons; he provides you with plenty of food and fills your hearts with joy.

PSALM 28:7—The LORD is my strength and my shield; my heart trusts in him, and I am helped. My heart leaps for joy and I will give thanks to him in song.

Anxiety, Worry, and Fear

Food is used to relax. In today's world, there are endless situations over which to worry. Psalm 139:23-24 says, "Search me, O God, and know my heart; test me and know my anxious thoughts. See if there is any offensive way in me, and lead me in the way everlasting." God knows if we are anxious! He wants us to stop feeling responsible and worried for those things we can't control. Jesus tells us not to worry even about our basic needs in life (Matthew 6:25-34).

Worry paralyzes our faith and draws our attention away from the faithfulness of God. Paul tells us to be anxious about nothing (Philippians 4:6) and then explains how we can accomplish this—by thanking God and sharing our concerns with Him through prayer. That is to be followed by meditating on God's goodness. The result is His supernatural peace resting on us.

Numerous times in the Bible we are told to hold fast against fear.

1 JOHN 4:18—There is no room in love for fear. Well-formed love banishes fear. Since fear is crippling, a fearful life—fear of death, fear of judgment—is one not yet fully formed in love. (MSG)

ISAIAH 35:4—Tell fearful souls, "Courage! Take heart! GOD is here, right here, on his way to put things right and redress all wrongs. He's on his way! He'll save you!" (MSG)

Disappointment/Hurt

There are so many opportunities to be disappointed with others that we could spend our whole lives eating in response to this one emotion. People make mistakes, betray us, are self-centered, and don't always look out for our best interests. Thus, our faith and confidence must be in the Lord. Even then, we may feel let down or hurt, even by God, and overeat as a result.

If this is the case, there is a problem of trust. He orders your steps and will allow difficulty in your life for a purpose. However, God's promise is to be with you through tough times. Focus on what you can learn from disappointment, but trust God to work it for your own good in His due time and in His way.

ISAIAH 26:3-4—You will keep in perfect peace him whose mind is steadfast, because he trusts in you. Trust in the LORD forever, for the LORD, the LORD, is the Rock eternal.

Emptiness

So many people go through life feeling empty and without purpose. Eating becomes a way to try and fill that empty place inside, but nothing will fill that void like an authentic relationship with God. He desires to draw close and be with you. He wants to fill you with good things and has a plan and purpose for you specifically. Engage with God in a new way. Be filled with His Word and when you feel empty, hunger and thirst for righteousness. His promise is that we will be filled if we "hunger and thirst for righteousness" (Matthew 5:6). We must fill the emptiness that only God can fill so that our lives are not controlled by our appetites for other things, because nothing but God can come close to fulfilling us. Emptiness leads us to fill our lives with everything but the one thing we truly need—God.

Procrastination

Eating is a great way to delay unpleasant tasks or to waste time. Perhaps you eat to avoid doing things you'd rather not do. But think about it! Has food ever made an unpleasant task go away? No! The task will still be there when you finish eating. It's best to tackle a task head-on, delegate it to someone else, or decide not to do the task at all.

Boredom

When there is nothing to do, eating is an activity that can fill time. Thinking about what you will eat next is a way of filling time that might otherwise be spent thinking of other unpleasant things. Food then becomes an obsession. If you are unsure how you would spend your time if you weren't eating, cooking, or planning meals, you may need to address this reason. Perhaps you will need to develop hobbies or find other ways to relax. For some people, this means trying new things and getting comfortable with relaxation.

Rejection

Food doesn't make rejection go away. Read this journal entry and see if it rings true for you.

The things I am learning about myself are incredible—specifically, why I have acted and/or reacted to people and situations the way I have. I realize that I have lived most of my life with a thick, protective bubble around myself. You know, the kind of person who has many casual friends, but hardly any close ones. The kind of person who seems really tough on the outside, but if you dig a little deeper, you find they aren't the person you first thought. I've also learned that even at 350 pounds, I was a marathon runner. Not the type of runner who wins races, but the type of runner who runs from people, churches, love, constructive criticism, and, if I'm really honest, reality.

In taking a closer look, I see that at a very young age I learned I couldn't trust people to love, protect, nurture, or even meet my most basic needs. When I tried to get these needs met by asking, I was repeatedly rejected. Even a small child will eventually stop asking for help if it means experiencing less pain for the moment. This pattern of rejection became a lifestyle. And, eventually, I found a substitute for these basic needs in my life. The substitute was food.

Praise God, the walls around me are beginning to fall. The thick protective bubble is thinning, and my run has slowed to a walk. I believe the Lord is going to heal me in these areas, and the root fear of rejection will no longer have a hold in my life.

—CATHY

Rejection is hard to handle whether you weigh 120 pounds or 300 pounds. It is especially difficult to swallow when it comes from those who are supposed to love us. One way to deal with rejection is to do what Cathy did—to try not to feel it and cover it up by eating. When people let you down, food can become your friend. It is always available, tastes good, and satisfies for the moment. But no matter how many times you shove a slice of pizza down your throat, the pain won't go away. The hurt still lingers beneath the layers of fat.

To be healed, you must face rejection. Feel it with all your soul. Pour out your heart to the Lord. Once you've allowed yourself to really feel the pain of rejection, pray and ask God to take it. Then, ask Christ to speak His truth to you. You see, the enemy uses emotional pain to implant lies—that no one will want or love you; that people will only hurt you; that if only you were thinner . . . all lies!

The truth is that there is someone who will never reject you and is completely trustworthy. Your acceptance has nothing to do with your actions or your weight. Jesus unconditionally loves you because you are His. Know that He identifies with your pain. According to Isaiah 53, Christ was despised, rejected, and a man of sorrow. Because of His great love for you, He suffered the pain of rejection and crucified it once and for all on the cross. Once you allow His truth to soak your spirit, you can give up the pain of rejection and accept God's unfailing love.

If you've suffered a number of rejections, try to understand that those people were probably not rejecting you personally as much as the concept of you or what you represented. If you suffered parental rejection, for example, your parents probably rejected the concept of having a child with needs, rather than rejecting you as an individual. Rejection still hurts, but it may be easier to forgive someone once you realize that person had problems of his/her own that were taken out on you. Whatever the case, you will need to forgive those who rejected you.

Loss of Control

Isn't it interesting that when we feel out of control, we eat out of control? We actually create the very thing we fear. We fear we'll lose control, so we try to control the people around us or our circumstances. Of course, we can't do that and end up feeling out of control and then stuff food inside. Here's the reality: If you think you have control, you need that red pill again. Control is elusive and no amount of eating will change that. You are not in control, so you might as well surrender to the One who is.

Express Your Feelings

Once you have identified your feelings, you must learn to express them directly rather than medicating them with food. Feelings can be expressed by talking them out to a friend, writing them in a journal like Cathy did, and/or by crying and giving direct vent to feelings. For example, you might say out loud, "I am so sad right now because I feel ignored." Give verbal expression to your feelings instead of swallowing them or stuffing them away. Allow yourself to feel whatever the feeling is until the intensity subsides. Then determine if there is a need behind the feeling, such as a need to be loved, accepted, approved of, or respected. Many times the urge to eat represents an unmet need. Get to the heart of the feeling and decide if you are being realistic. If you must grieve a loss or work on ways to get your needs met, don't eat to feel better. Deal with the feelings.

Confession—Good for the Soul

Once you become more comfortable identifying feelings and allowing yourself to feel them, you need to be honest about what is going on inside of you. There is sickness in secrecy. The sinning Psalmist said, "When I kept silent, my bones wasted away . . ." (32:3). When we are willing to be open, healing becomes possible. By breaking our silence and speaking the truth about ourselves aloud to another person, we move out of the darkness and bring secrets into the light. Confessing our sins and talking about the wrongs done to us is another key to spiritual healing and health.

It is clearly important to God that men and women verbally express the struggles hidden in their hearts. Verbalization gives substance to inarticulate thoughts, and words affirm the realities of which we have become aware. Even on the key issue of Christian salvation, belief is to be affirmed with spoken words. Paul wrote, "If you confess with your mouth, 'Jesus is Lord,' and believe in your heart that God raised him from the dead, you will be saved. For it is with your heart that you believe and are justified, and it is with your mouth that you confess and are saved" (Romans 10:9-10).

Unexpressed thoughts do not allow others to give input or challenge us to see the truth. When we confess our thoughts, we put others in the position of advising us, praying for us, and sharing our struggles. We must be careful however; confession requires confidentiality. It is an invitation to intimacy and involves trust in both God and another person—a trust that is absolutely necessary for us to be able to truly reveal our secrets.

Openness is an outward act of trust that enables us to cleanse our souls from the inside out. If you want to break free from emotional eating, you must confess the need that is not being met and be honest about what you truly feel. Pretending not to have anger or not to be jealous will not help you heal, but honesty brings about authentic change. Confession means we:

- submit ourselves to God's ways of handling secrets.
- are willing to overcome our fear of rejection by revealing our failures to another person and admitting we need help from fellow believers.
- reject our habit of self-protective secretiveness.
- admit to at least one other person that we have fallen short of God's best, be it through character defects or judgment errors.
- stop trying to mask our true feelings and put our vague sense of guilt into written or spoken words, without making excuses.

By openly confessing our flaws and struggles, there is hope for healing. Admit what you really feel and where you struggle emotionally. Come out of the eating closet and identify your hurts and losses. Do what James 5:16 commands: "Confess your sins to each other and pray for each other so that you can live together whole and healed" (MSG).

Have more than one person to talk to about your struggles so you don't overburden a person. Also, you won't feel guilty asking for help multiple times if you can spread around the need. Find someone who is a good listener, humble, trustworthy, evidences a quiet godliness, and is stable and positive. You want to avoid people with personal agendas, controlling personalities, or those who are needy, unstable, or sexually attractive to you. If you are married, it's better to find a same sex confidante so that sexual tension will not be an issue. Lastly, remember to treat this person as a friend, not a therapist.

Keep a Prayer Journal

We also recommend keeping a prayer journal, a tool to help document prayer requests and answers to prayer. They also are an excellent way to track your emotional swings. Whatever you feel, take it to God in prayer. Don't edit your feelings; just record them honestly. If you aren't sure how to begin, use this format and try this meaningful exercise:

1. Spend time in the Word or a devotional reading.
2. Write down a key verse or main idea from the reading.
3. Write out your prayer requests in response to what you have read.
4. Spend time in prayer.
5. Wait for a personal word from the Lord. (This step takes time to develop.) Wait before the Lord in silence and allow Him to speak to you. Then write down what you believe you hear in your spirit. Don't be surprised if you think you don't hear anything at first. Most people report that it takes time to learn how to be quiet before the Lord and listen for His voice. With time, you will develop your spiritual hearing.

Substitute a New Behavior for Eating

Pain is not optional, but misery is. You can't always control pain, but you can do something about misery. If you are looking for a quick fix to emotional pain, you're reading the wrong book! Healing is often progressive because it requires changes in your character and actions. The way you cope with emotional pain must change if you decide to no longer eat your way through it.

Keeping a record of what you do when you become emotionally upset is a good way to watch your progress—perhaps in a journal. The journey to finding new alternatives to eating might look like this:

Event: Received an upsetting phone call from my ex
Emotion: Very hurt
Reaction: Went to the refrigerator and opened the door to eat

Now, think of a new way to cope with that feeling. What could you substitute for eating?

New Reaction: Call a friend and let her pray with me

Here's another example:

Event: Heard someone gossip about me at church
Emotion: Anger
Reaction: Stopped for fries at a fast food restaurant
New Reaction: Gently confront the person who did the gossiping

To help yourself choose alternatives to eating, make a list of twenty behaviors you can substitute for eating the next time an intense emotion triggers that desire. Your list should include things you can do while driving, being at home, at work, or on the go. Post the list on your refrigerator and make a copy to take with you. Every time you are tempted to eat because you feel an unpleasant emotion, pull out your list and choose a new thing to do. Feel free to borrow ideas from this list:

· Take a short walk and cool down.

· Listen to calming music.

· Take three deep breaths.

· Distract yourself with something in the room or car.

· Take a bubble bath.

· Call a friend.

· Count to 20.

· Take a short nap.

· Pray and ask God to help you.

· Turn up the radio and get lost in the music.

· Stand up and do some stretches.

· Go to the bathroom, even if it's only to splash water on your face.

· Play with your dog.

· Play with your child.

· Watch a funny movie.

· Go somewhere quiet and practice deep muscle relaxation.

· Clean something.

· Run up and down the stairs to release tension.

· Work on a crossword puzzle.

· Play a video game.

March 29, 2004—Incredible! I just made it through an entire week in which food has not been an issue. I'm serious! I haven't wasted one minute wondering what I'm going to have for dinner the next day. I haven't been secretly imagining what unhealthy food snacks I'd devour if no one was around to see me. Food just hasn't been the primary thing on my mind. I even went to New York this weekend just for fun. I had a blast doing the whole tourist thing, and it wasn't about the food. I never thought this could be possible. I feel like the food handcuffs have somehow been released, and I'm now a free woman. Praise God for weeks like this. —CATHY

Maybe you've been hurt by a cruel divorce, an abusive father, a betraying friend, or an insulting boss. Whatever the cause of your hurt, it's time to stop using food as an emotional crutch and let the pain surface. When you do, you might experience intense feelings of anger or fear, but there will not be healing until you face those feelings.

Just let the feelings come, and ask God to help you understand exactly why you feel as you do. Don't try to edit your thoughts. Whatever comes in to your mind, grab that thought. Most likely it is a lie that was implanted at the time of the emotional pain when you first experienced those feelings. Try to identify the lie, and once you find it, ask Jesus to speak His truth to you. Wait and listen for His voice, whether it comes in the form of a whisper of His Spirit or a visual picture He may give you. Wait on Him and expect Him to bring truth. His truth brings release from that lie.

If you continue to take every hurt and pain to Christ, lay them at His feet, and refuse to believe the lies, the food handcuffs will drop off you just like they did for Cathy. Come out of the eating closet. Exchange it for a prayer closet—a place filled with peace and rest.

8
—— Changing the Viewing ——

Have you seen the reality television show called *Extreme Makeover?* The concept of the show is this: Each week, the producers present the viewing audience with two or more people who are extremely insecure about their looks. Because of their physical flaws, they lack confidence, become introverts, and/or don't fully engage in life. For years they have suffered teasing and insults concerning their appearances. Their stories touch us—we feel for them. Some of us can even relate to their emotional pain.

People write to the show and pitch their reasons for needing a makeover. When chosen, they react with delight, knowing they've basically won the makeover lottery—in the form of top plastic surgeons, dentists, eye surgeons, fashion experts, hair stylists, makeup artists, and personal trainers, all contributing to the extreme makeover. With a promise of life transformation in just six weeks, those chosen consent to going under the plastic surgery knife.

As they choose their new bodies, they can be sculpted to new proportions—breast implants, liposuction, a chin implant, face-lift, rhinoplasty, corrective eye surgery, even new dentures. If they want it, they get it!

As we watch these people anxiously go into surgery and then recovery, the emotional buildup begins. Soon their lives will be dramatically altered. We become voyeurs to the process. It's like watching a butterfly emerge from a cocoon as the metamorphosis takes approximately six weeks. At the end of that time, a limousine escorts the new person back to the reality of their life and family. And in true Hollywood fashion, their coming-out party happens on a stage amid lights and cameras. The audience gasps with awe, applauds, cries, and hugs. The difference is dramatic and a testimony to the power of an extreme makeover.

All that to say, though we certainly feel sorrow for the emotional pain those chosen few have endured because of their appearances, the message is disconcerting. The solution proffered—that being thin and beautiful will fix life's problems—only adds to the obsession our culture has with the body. Record numbers of people in bondage to eating disorders, as well as most Americans who are unhappy with their bodies, are embracing this message. If life's problems can be fixed with surgery, why shouldn't we all go under the knife? Pretty soon none of us will measure up!

The television show has the right idea, but the wrong solution. The truth is, we all need an extreme makeover. If you struggle with negative self-image, the solution is surgery within the heart. The results last a lifetime, and the transformation that comes from being the bride of Christ is beyond any physical makeover one could ever experience. It is extreme, life changing, and affirming—"But we all, with unveiled face, beholding as in a mirror the glory of the Lord, are being transformed into the same image from glory to glory, just as by the Spirit of the Lord" (2 Corinthians 3:18 NKJV). Now that's an extreme makeover we want to support!

How does such a makeover happen? One important step in the process is the renewing of your mind, or, as we like to call it, *changing the viewing* in the way you think about yourself, God, and others. To start, let us address these three key areas.

Body Image

Whose image do you reflect? Should you try to meet society's warped standards of beauty and fitness, or should you be content with the body you were given while making every effort to be in good health? In Genesis 1:26-27, God explains that we are made in His image and reflect His likeness. He declared His created design "good," meaning that nothing about our bodies is a mistake. However, by not taking care of our bodies, we do harm. Eating too much food and not getting enough exercise are actually abuses against the human body that are a direct result of the human will. As a result, the body should not be viewed as the enemy in this weight loss journey.

Identity

Your acceptance, security, and significance are to be found in Christ. If you look to any other source for your true identity, you'll be disappointed by the result. The root of all image problems is related to identity. Your identity must be fully secure in Christ. You are one of His and must not allow yourself to be defined otherwise.

Worth

God's love for you has nothing to do with your appearance or weight. You are His beautiful bride and are valued and esteemed *because of Him,* not because of the way you look. He looks at your heart and wants to capture it. You were bought with a price: the precious blood of the Lamb. Value is determined by how much someone is willing to pay for it. Christ obviously values you a great deal in that He gave His life for you.

Your perspective regarding your body, identity, and worth may require new focus as you meditate on God's Word and learn more specifically how God thinks about you. If you doubt these truths, then your mind is in need of renewal. As you make changes in eating and exercise, you must also focus on becoming a person of spiritual beauty—one who imitates Christ and desires to be like Him in mind, body, and spirit.

A New Thought

When my (Dr. Linda's) daughter was young, she asked me an interesting question that really got me thinking. As she watched me step out of the shower and towel off the excess water one morning, she just stared at me. Thinking deeply (or as deep as a five-year-old can think), she asked, "Mom, will I get that crinkly stuff on your legs? It doesn't look too good."

I almost fell over. This tiny child was staring at my cellulite! And her conclusion was that it didn't look "too good." Well, I knew this was an important mother-daughter moment that could influence her feelings about her own body in years to come. So I calmly looked at my cellulite (that act in itself is a miracle) and explained, "You won't get this crinkly stuff on your legs until you are my age. And when you do, it's no big deal. It's just crinkly stuff." Part of me believed what I was saying, but the other part was screaming, "Oh really, no big deal? How long did you obsess over your thighs before you came to accept them?"[65]

Fortunately, by this point in my life, the cellulite wasn't a big deal. Years ago, my answer would have been different. I, like so many men and women, had to learn to make peace with my physical body. No matter what size we are, accepting our bodies is not easy to do in this culture.

We never measure up to the ideals plastered on billboards, magazines, commercials, and movies. And seeing images of perfection day in and day out does a number on our thinking. From Botox to cellulite creams, the message is that you can never be too thin, too fit, or too perfect. Yet it's time for all of us to think twice about these messages, because they have serious impact on our lives as well as others.

One of the best sensations I (Steve) have ever had is the feeling of weightlessness experienced on a wild ride called the Fire Ball. In between the soaring up and plummeting down, something amazing happens. For about two seconds you are up and out of your seat and held into the contraption only by a harness. Literally, you are floating in a state of weightlessness. And what a feeling of freedom and joy that brings!

This is what I want for you. I want you to wake up in the morning and not have to drag yourself out of bed; to not have one thought about your weight or feeling about who you are relating to your weight. You would know your weight but it would not define you. You would not feel too heavy or too light or too anything. You would be able to relate without worrying about something being too big or bulging or even what others were thinking about your appearance. Your life would be something beyond weight, size, and comparison. You would be free. You would be weightless.

Negative body image is like a modern day plague that continues to torment us. But it doesn't have to be. We can resist cultural prescriptions and renew our minds with biblical thought. Our bodies are the dwelling place of the Holy Spirit (1 Corinthians 3:16), literally holy temples!

There is a healthy balance between body obsession and hating our bodies. Somewhere in the middle is acceptance and responsibility. The way we think about our bodies will be reflected externally. Proverbs 23:7 says, "For as he thinks in his heart, so is he" (NKJV). Hence, you are what you think! When a person hates their body, you can tell by the way he or she talks about it. Yet to hate your body is to reject the beautiful creation God has made in His image. Instead, you must accept your body, flaws and all, and take care for that holy temple. Five key steps to accepting your body are:

1. STOP DEGRADING YOUR BODY. "I am so fat. Who would want me?" "I'm ugly and undesirable." These kinds of statements are highly negative and lead to negative feelings. You would not say such things about a friend, and you shouldn't talk about yourself this way either. Become your best encourager rather than worst critic. That voice would say, "You are overweight, but you're working on it."

2. STOP PUTTING LIFE ON HOLD BECAUSE YOU DON'T LIKE YOUR BODY. Dive in and do what you love to do. Feel good knowing that you are making every effort you can to change your weight, while accepting that your body is the Holy Spirit's temple no matter what and a reflection of God's likeness. Live in the present reality as you implement changes for the future.

3. THINK OF GOOD THINGS TO SAY ABOUT YOURSELF. You are more than your weight. Focus on the positive qualities you have outside of your physical size. We are not asking you to boast, but do become more balanced and realistic. We all have good qualities that can be emphasized.

4. DEVELOP YOUR OWN STYLE AND PERSONALITY. Not everyone judges you by your weight. Take a chance and reach out to others rather than hiding behind your weight. Let your true personality shine.

5. GET YOUR ESTEEM FROM GOD. Self-esteem is a misleading term. None of us can truly have esteem by looking to the *self.* The *self* is sinful, self-centered, and easily deceived. God esteems you just because He chose and loves you. You don't have to earn His esteem. You already have it. Remember, He values you so much that He gave His only Son to die for you.

Thoughts lead to feelings. Feelings lead to actions. Actions influence our perceptions, which then influence our thoughts. It's a vicious cycle. What we think affects how we feel, which in turn can prompt us to eat in response. Thus, many negative feelings can be avoided by changing the thought that prompts the feeling. If, for example, I feel sad because I purposefully think, *Nobody cares about me*, I can change my sad feeling by changing the thought to a more positive and realistic one—*God cares about me even when others don't*. Since this thought is reassuring and doesn't make me feel sad, I am unlikely to eat as a response to it.

If we apply the RISE formula to our thoughts, here are our goals:

REDUCE: negative thoughts and self-degrading statements.
INCREASE: your awareness of God; esteem and acceptance of the body you were given.
SUBSTITUTE: positive thoughts for negative ones and a view of yourself that is not defined by your weight.
ELIMINATE: thinking errors and lies.

Renewing the Mind

In this context, the word "renew" means a change of heart and life. It is work the Holy Spirit does in us. As we offer our bodies as a living sacrifice to God, we allow the Holy Spirit to radically work in our hearts and minds. Renewing the mind is different from positive thinking in that truth must be experienced from the One who is truth.

Whenever something negative or traumatic happens to us, the enemy uses those circumstances to implant a lie, because his plan is to deceive us about who God is. During times of emotional pain, he tries hard to seduce us away from God's truth and into a pit of darkness. If we don't know the truth, or we let our spiritual guard down, we can accept his lies in place of truth, just as Eve did.

So much of the pain and turmoil we feel today has to do with lies implanted from times when we experienced hurt and were wounded. Many of us continue to struggle with overeating because we believe a host of lies. We believe we are hopeless, that God doesn't care, that people are always letting us down. And though none of these statements is true, we adjust our reality to make them true.

While we are saved and our spirits are made new in Christ (2 Corinthians 5:17), our minds are still in need of renewal. Yet we cannot be free of the lies and distorted thinking on our own power. A renewed mind comes as we receive truth from Christ and deeply plant His Word in our hearts.

How many times have you known something to be true, such as, "God loves me and would never leave me," and yet you *feel* this isn't true. Your experience tells you that what you know to be true isn't true. And here is the great disconnect: We can know truth in our heads but not have it connect to our hearts. We need an experience of truth to make it real to us and connect our heads and hearts. That's where prayer comes in. When you know your heart says one thing and your head says another, ask Christ to speak His truth to you. Read His Word and ask Him to penetrate it deep into your mind and soul. Look at the Gospels. Do you notice that Jesus healed (an experience) and then spoke to the person (cognitive)? The Truth gave truth, both experientially and cognitively.

Identify the lies that create your emotional pain. Lies can come to us by the words of others, by our own perceptions, or during times of hurt and trauma. Once you identify a lie, ask Christ to speak His truth. Here's an example: An obese woman struggled with urges to binge regularly. In counseling, she discussed times she was prevented from having food as a form of punishment when she was a child. The lie she believed was that she would never get enough food. Thus she binged because she was afraid food would not be available. And though she knew in her head that this wasn't true, she prayed and asked God to show her His truth. She describes hearing Christ tell her that He always has enough of what she needs. She reads scriptures that remind her of this truth and meditates on them. As soon as she did this, that lie no longer had power over her. Experientially, she knew her needs would be met.

In another case, a man was deeply hurt over the rejection from his wife when she divorced him. As a result, he began to think he was unlovable. Those in the adult singles' group at his church encouraged him to join the group. He did and found people willing to accept him and spend time with him. His experience with this group of believers countered his earlier belief. "If these people can accept me, and I know God accepts me, maybe I'm not unlovable." The power of the lie was broken through the development of a new community. His overeating diminished when he was no longer eating out of feelings of rejection.

Perhaps the biggest lie we tell ourselves is that all we can do about our problem is to pray to God to get rid of it. And though this might be true, and you can pray that prayer, the answer is often going to require more than waiting for God. Or God may choose not to take away this burden, which is often the case.

Whether or not you have a life of meaning and purpose or stagnation and death is quite often dependent on what we are willing to change. We wait for God to do what God is waiting for us to do. Why? Because God wants to build our character, and the way He does that is by sticking with us through a struggle, gently supporting our efforts if they are honorable and glorify Him.

Take the Negative Thought Captive

In 2 Corinthians 10:5 we are told to take our thoughts captive. "We use our powerful God-tools for smashing warped philosophies, tearing down barriers erected against the truth of God, fitting every loose thought and emotion and impulse into the structure of life shaped by Christ" (MSG).

If you grew up in a home in which you were constantly criticized, negative thoughts have been deeply ingrained. Don't worry. You can renew your mind with the help of God and others.

To apply this Scripture, we must be aware of what we are thinking. Once we realize the thought is negative, self-degrading, or untrue, we should stop the thought. To stop a thought, pretend you are grabbing it out of the air. You have now taken it captive. You say, "I've got you, thought. Now what am I going to do with you?" Hopefully, you will smash it or replace it with a thought that is true, one that fits a life shaped by Christ.

Here's an example of this principle in action. The thought occurs: *I just ate all those cookies. I am so bad.* The latter part of that thought must be stopped. Grab it and replace it with God's truth by saying, "I am not bad. Christ is in me, and though I am tempted and do sin, when this happens I ask for forgiveness and move on. I wish I didn't eat all those cookies, but it's not the end of the world. I can regain control right now with God's help. Lord, give me the self-control I need right now."

In order to lose it for life, you have to gain control of your thoughts. And with practice, you can do this. Sometimes it helps to put a rubber band on your wrist and snap it every time you tell yourself a negative thought or lie. The mild pain is a simple reminder to grab the negative thought. Until you do something like this, you may not realize how many times a day negative thoughts race through your mind. Like spam mail on a computer, the thoughts just show up and keep on coming. As with e-mail, the trick is to not click on the thoughts to open them. Instead, delete them instantly and avoid giving negative thoughts a foothold in your mind, because they are the messages of Satan, not God.

Keep a Thought Record

A tool that is often used to help people get in touch with their thoughts is the Dysfunctional Thought Record (DTR).[66] This is a simple chart laid out as follows (see Appendix F):

Dysfunctional Thought Record

Date	Situation	Emotion/ Intensity	Automatic Thought	Rational Response/ Intensity	Outcome
3-20	Overate	Disgust / 80%	I am a loser	I blew it but I can get back on track / 10%	

Here's how you use the chart. You record the date and briefly describe the situation. Next write down what emotion you felt and rate its intensity from 0-100 percent in terms of emotional intensity. Then record the automatic thought that came into your mind. Once you identify the automatic thought and write it down, try to think of a more rational and true thought and write it down. Then re-rate your emotion. It should be less intense.

Keeping this chart will help you recognize the thoughts that cue your emotions. And you can review your thoughts and write alternative ways to think about the situation. For example, let's use the situation of overeating. The emotion recorded is *disgust* and you gave it an 80 percent rating, which means you felt it intensely. Your automatic thought was, *I am a loser.* The more rational response or truth is, *I blew it but can get back on track. It was only ten cookies. I am weak in my own power, but with Christ I can do all things.* You re-rate your emotion to 10 percent.

Eventually, you'll be able to do this exercise in your head. The purpose is to expose the automatic, negative thoughts and replace them with more rational alternative thoughts that are consistent with biblical truth.

The Answer for Anxious Thoughts

"I am just anxious; I'm not thinking anything." Wrong! You have thoughts behind those anxious feelings. The feelings may be so intense that you aren't aware of the self-talk that preceded your anxiety, but such talk is behind most anxious feelings. Remember, your thoughts impact your feelings.

Most anxious people think, *What if...?* We suggest you change the "What if..." to "So what ..." to reduce anxiety. Does this sound easy? It's not. Anxious thoughts are automatic for people with anxiety problems. A person may *feel* anxious and yet be unaware of preceding thoughts. The first step is to identify your thought before the anxious feeling occurs, although the thought won't always be obvious. For example, Pat sat in a meeting with several of his superiors. He was nervous about his presentation and flashed back to a time early on in his career when he botched a presentation. These thoughts started running through Pat's head: *What if I mess up again? I could get fired. I will embarrass myself.* The more Pat allowed himself to think these thoughts, the more anxious he became. By the time he stood up to give his presentation, he was close to panic. Had this man used his self-talk in a positive way, he might have warded off anxiety. *I may have messed up early on in my career, but now I'm much more experienced. I've done these presentations many times with good outcomes. I have every reason to believe these people will like what I have to say and be impressed.*

Notice how the first self-talk creates or reinforces anxious feelings while the second example dismisses anxious thoughts and builds confidence. Self-talk is that powerful. When lies and negative thoughts become frequent and a regular part of your thinking, they create and sustain anxiety, which is often responded to by overeating. Anxious people think in ways that perpetuate anxiety. Review this checklist and find out if you think like an anxious person.

Am I Anxious?

○ ***It's going to be a catastrophe!*** *You think of the most extreme negative consequences possible and assume it's going to happen. Disaster will hit whether it's in the form of an event or personal humiliation and embarrassment.*

○ ***It's personal!*** *Whatever happens around you is somehow personally relevant to you and will most likely happen to you next. For example, if there is a fire in the city, your house is next.*

○ ***It could happen!*** *Here's why. You magnify the one part of the issue that could create a problem and ignore the non-threatening parts. For example, you forget the words to the song you've practiced multiple times. Even though it's unlikely, since you've never forgotten the words during practice before, you tell yourself it could happen.*

○ ***It doesn't matter what else is going on. I see danger.*** *You ignore the context of a problem and choose to focus on the one thing that could be dangerous or problematic. For example, your daughter could fall off the swing even though the grass is soft, the swing almost touches the ground, and she loves to be outside. Anxious thinkers focus on the possibility of falling off the swing even though the likelihood of harm is slight.*

○ ***I can tell this is trouble!*** *At any sign of trouble, you immediately jump to conclusions. For example, air turbulence means the plane is crashing. Or a tightness in your chest means you are dying from a heart attack. A call from the school means your child is in trouble.*

○ ***I can't. I don't have what it takes. I won't be able to do it.*** *You believe nothing will change and you can't meet the challenge. You have given up* *before starting and aren't asking God to help you overcome your weakness. Though you can't do something in your own power, God can do all things through you if you allow His power to be made known.*

○ **It will happen again.** *Because something happened once, you assume it will happen again. You overgeneralize to the next situation. For instance, you panicked the last time you saw your ex-husband and assume you will panic every time you see him in the future.*

○ **It's all or nothing.** *All-or-nothing thinking is just like it sounds. You believe things happen all the time or not at all. Your color perspective includes two colors: black and white. But definitely not gray! All-or-nothing thinkers are often disappointed and need to build tolerance for failure and imperfection. Any "mistake" has the potential to be thought of as a catastrophe, which will possibly lead to overeating and thoughts of failure.*

○ **It's perfection that's required.** *These two phrases play over and over in your mind—I should have, or I have to . . . You are the classic perfectionist who always falls short of the job and worries about your failures. These thoughts don't allow for mistakes or human fallibility.*

○ **It's going to be bad.** *You are far too critical and need to give yourself a break! You need a shot of God-esteem. Your classic thoughts are:* I can't believe I did that. How stupid. What an idiot I am.

○ **What about . . . ?** *You are the classic worrier. Nothing can happen without you fearing all the possibilities for disaster or problems. You fail to recognize that you really don't have control. Worrying about everything that can go wrong is sin. God tells us to be anxious about nothing. He wants us to hand over the worry to Him. He will take care of us no matter what.*

If you relate to these statements, you need to change out your thoughts. Write down positive statements that will counter the negative ones, and use scriptures to back up your new positions. For example, instead of thinking, *I can't do that because it's too scary,* tell yourself: *It looks scary but I can meet a new challenge. The worst possible thing that can happen is that I'll feel scared for a moment and then it will pass. And if I make it through, I will have accomplished something new.*

After you've written down positive statements to replace your negative thoughts, meditate on the truth. Here's a powerful scripture you can always use: "I can do everything through him who gives me strength" (Philippians 4:13). The next time you feel anxious, stop and ask yourself what thought is making you feel worried. Chances are it's a negative thought that needs changing.

Acknowledging the possibility of danger in a situation does not necessarily make you an anxious person. You may be a realist. But if your focus is constantly on the possible harm, or the one factor that could go wrong, or whether you did the right thing, you are an anxious thinker. Anxious thinking makes anxious people, but by changing your thoughts, you can lessen your anxiety and even the feelings that result from the thought.

Changing the Attitude

It's 5:30 a.m. The alarm goes off and Rita rolls out of bed. Exhausted from the night before, Rita forces her body to head to the shower. As she towels off, her daily fight with anxiety begins. Every morning she spends four hours getting ready for work. Every hair must be perfectly in place and her makeup impeccable.

Rita worries that people will reject her if she appears less than perfect. Even though she knows her thoughts and behaviors are irrational, she can't stop herself from performing the lengthy routine.

Worry is Rita's constant companion. It helps her prepare for unpredictable moments in life. Her greatest fear is that she will somehow be rejected for the way she looks. To change this irrational behavior, Rita had to be convinced that her worry was unproductive and not helping her control anything. In fact, the worry was controlling her. It was time to say goodbye to her lifelong friend—worry.

In order to stop worrying, she had to change her attitude by embracing two ideas: First, her sacrifice of time and energy was not worth the small amount of control she thought she gained, because uncertainty is part of the world in which we live. People can reject her for all sorts of reasons, including her weight. So rather than avoid this uncertainty, Rita needed to accept it as a part of her life.

Second, Rita needed to accept that this type of comfort is overrated. All of Rita's hours of makeup application were directed at making her feel more comfortable with her physical appearance. Now, comfort could no longer be the goal. Instead, she had to get comfortable with discomfort. She could learn to live with it, even if sometimes it was difficult or might feel lousy. But she needed to tolerate "lousy" and get past it.

When Rita allowed herself to feel discomfort, we applauded her and welcomed her to the human race. And we encouraged her to stay with the race and not run away from it! So every day, she was to wake up and recite this message:

Worry is unproductive. I can't predict how life will go today and that is OK. Discomfort will come, but it will also pass. I can live with uncertainty and change because God is in control, and He promises He won't give me anything I can't handle.

As Rita developed a new attitude about worry, her anxiety lifted. Gradually she cut down her morning routine to a reasonable time. To her amazement, it didn't seem to make any difference to her coworkers. When something felt out of Rita's control, she would check her thoughts by telling herself, "This is normal. Life is unpredictable. God will give me the grace to deal with it." Of course, the side effect was that Rita had more control over her eating.

Contain Stressful Thoughts

Stress can originate from your thoughts. Two good strategies to help with stressful thoughts are visualizing and meditation. We are not talking about repeating mantras or engaging in transcendental meditation, so please stay with us. Christians can meditate and visualize. The Bible even directs us to do so: "Whatever is true, whatever is noble, whatever is right, whatever is pure, whatever is lovely, whatever is admirable—if anything is excellent or praiseworthy—think about such things" (Philippians 4:8).

All you do is focus your mind on what brings you peace and a sense of well-being. Think about God's intense love for you and dedicate some time to Him. When we pray and spend time with our heavenly Father, we feel better and less stressed. This Dad has promised to take care of us and meet our needs. If that reality doesn't lessen your stress, nothing will!

Another tactic is to visualize yourself in a quiet, peaceful place. This is calming. Some people like to imagine themselves resting on a sunny beach with a gentle breeze, the smell of the ocean, clear skies, and water all present in their imagination. Other people find a mountain cabin in the snow to be a quiet, calming place.

Others imagine basking eternally in the presence of Christ. I (Dr. Linda) like to read Revelation 21 and picture the New Jerusalem based on the visual description John gives in that chapter—the gates, the angels, the gems, but mostly the glory of God that will shine and illuminate the city! It doesn't matter what scene you choose, as long as you think of something peaceful and try to engage all your senses in the scene. If you succeed, your anxious thoughts will melt as you settle into a place of peace.

True peace comes from having a personal relationship with Jesus Christ. One of His promises is to keep us in perfect peace if we keep our mind fixed on Him (Isaiah 26:3). God is the author of peace and serenity. Think about Him and His goodness, love, and all that He has done for you and will do as we approach His eternal presence.

A renewed mind is a mind that agrees with God. God is incapable of having bad motivations toward us, and yet we often attribute these to God. In Him, there is no darkness. When we know His character, His promises, and we believe who He says He is, we cannot think of God as bad or unloving. The key is intimacy with Him. The more you know Him, the more you trust and believe that He is truth. And the more time you spend with Him, the more you experience His truth.

In 2 Corinthians 1:8-9, Paul affirms that God brings comfort in the midst of trouble:

> We don't want you in the dark, friends, about how hard it was when all this came down on us in Asia province. It was so bad we didn't think we were going to make it. We felt like we'd been sent to death row; that it was all over for us. As it turned out, it was the best thing that could have happened. Instead of trusting in our own strength or wits to get out of it, we were forced to trust God totally—not a bad idea since he's the God who raises the dead! (MSG)

As you engage in the process to lose it for life, you will hit bumps along the way related to how you think. Sometimes we think too much! It is easy to question God in times of difficulty. We can grow impatient and allow the enemy to gain ground in our thoughts. But God wants to teach us to depend on Him all the time as we renew our minds with His truth and know that He is powerful and able to accomplish much in us if we submit to His plan.

9
Changing the Doing

Ever noticed how good intentions don't always bring success? The reality is that action is required to achieve goals. Knowing what we know about eating, exercising, and losing weight, we often try to will ourselves to do what is "right" and stay on our plan. Yet too often, we find ourselves doing what is wrong.

Faith is the belief or confidence that God will do all He says He will do. As we read God's Word and implant it deep into our hearts, action must follow what we read and hear. James confirms this in his epistle (1:22-25):

> Don't fool yourself into thinking that you are a listener when you are anything but, letting the Word go in one ear and out the other. Act on what you hear! Those who hear and don't act are like those who glance in the mirror, walk away, and two minutes later have no idea who they are, what they look like. But whoever catches a glimpse of the revealed counsel of God—the free life!—even out of the corner of his eye, and sticks with it, is no distracted scatterbrain but a man or woman of action. That person will find delight and affirmation in the action. (MSG)

Don't you want to be that person who finds delight and affirmation in action? With the Holy Spirit operating in your life, you are empowered to do those things you know to be true. Even if you have a history of weight loss failure, it's time to look forward and begin applying action to your decision to lose it for life. There is no time like the present to begin. God has already given you what you need to overcome. When you confess Christ as your Savior, the Holy Spirit takes up residence in you. It is His presence that empowers each of us to overcome.

Tools for Change

Change is a process that involves multiple steps. Below is an outline of six steps necessary to bring change to your life.

Illumination

When you see the need for change, you have reached illumination. It is, to be precise, your "light-bulb" moment—the point at which you finally understand your situation in a whole new way. As Ephesians 5:8 says, "You groped your way through that murk once, but no longer. You're out in the open now. The bright light of Christ makes your way plain. So no more stumbling around. Get on with it!" (MSG). Hopefully at this point in the program, your weaknesses have come to light and you are ready to get on with it.

Inspiration

Once you see the need for change, you must be inspired to make necessary changes. Ask God for His help and guidance. Change may be needed in several areas of your life—eating, exercise, dealing with your emotions, or how you think and act. Also ask God for the courage to change and be transformed into what is God's best for you. See what you can become and become motivated by the vision.

Examination

As we are inspired to make changes, we must take a good hard look at how we measure up to God's standards. Socrates once said, "An unexamined life is not worth living."[67] We couldn't agree more. How does your life measure up to God's standards? Do you imitate Christ in all you do? Are you living a holy life? Are you obedient to the Word? Whatever your answers are to these questions, the good news is you can begin today to evaluate your life according to God's Word. No one is perfect, but after examining your life closely, you should be more inclined to want to live in obedience to God's Word.

Motivation

Are you motivated to be used by God and to know His purposes for your life? When you understand that the life God has for you is beyond what you could even imagine, you have reached the step of motivation. Walking in His truth and staying obedient to His Word are your secret weapons to developing a purpose-driven life. God doesn't want you immobilized by your weight. Ask the Holy Spirit to fill you so full of Him that something beyond yourself will happen.

The more we seek the kingdom of God and all His righteousness first, the more used of God we will be. Colossians 3:12 tells us how to "dress" for this type of success—"So, chosen by God for this new life of love, dress in the wardrobe God picked out for you: compassion, kindness, humility, quiet strength, discipline" (MSG).

If you have struggled with motivation for years, perhaps it is time to realize that you just don't have the ability to motivate yourself. But you can reach out to someone else; you can bring people around you to help coach you and provide you with the motivation you do not possess on your own. This is what God has in mind when we surround ourselves with a body of believers.

Determination

No matter what you've been through already, don't give up. If you fall down and blow it, get up and try again. God gives us second chances. He wants us to succeed. With Christ, all things are possible. Stay in the fight and keep reaching for the prize.

All the people I know who have lost weight and kept it off have had a tremendous amount of determination. They just won't give up. If their weight plateaus, they just keep doing what they have been doing while making minor changes that eventually result in a return of weight loss. For them, there is no excuse good enough to give up, so they persevere. And the longer they stay determined, the stronger their transformation becomes.

Realization

Supernatural things can happen. Persevere until change comes, and be of good courage. You are a champion because of God's ability to change people. Your life matters and God has plans for you. James 1:12 says, "Blessed is the man who perseveres under trial, because when he has stood the test, he will receive the crown of life that God has promised to those who love him."

Continue to RISE Above the Challenges

You will want to review the RISE formula from each chapter and make changes in your eating and exercise habits, as well as how you deal with your emotions and thinking. Spiritually, the more you press into God and depend on Him, the better you'll do as you lose it for life.

Let's revisit our RISE formula again in terms of behavior:

REDUCE: eating in response to social cues.

INCREASE: the number of changes you make. Start small and add more as you are able.

Substitute: forgiveness for any bitterness or unresolved misdeed; new behaviors for eating.

Eliminate: eating for the wrong reasons.

Reduce

Another type of cue besides those based on emotions or feelings that often trigger overeating is a social cue. One of the most common social triggers is the television commercial. Visually, TV commercials stimulate our desire to eat. The best way to handle commercials, especially late at night when you are tired and your defenses are down, is to use the remote to click past the commercials. Don't watch them and you won't be drawn in by the trigger. And certainly don't watch food channels or cooking shows! Both can trigger a desire to overeat.

Another common social cue that triggers eating is driving in the car. If you are used to downing Big Gulps, eating candy bars, or running by the drive-thru for a quick pick-me-up snack, you have conditioned yourself to eat in the car. Food billboards can also stimulate the urge to eat. This association of the car with eating must be broken. We know the concept sounds impossible, but the best way to do this is to not eat in the car at all, even though eating in the car is almost an American way of life! However, if you stop doing this, you'll not only reduce your calorie intake, but also have a cleaner car! Relegate all eating to the kitchen table.

What about the movies? Do you have to have that buttered popcorn to watch a movie? We hear your emphatic YES—because a movie just wouldn't be a movie without popcorn or the super-sized Junior Mints™, right? Surprise! Movies can be very enjoyable without the snacks. Drink a full glass of water before you go, and eat a low-calorie snack so the sight and smell of all those goodies won't be so tempting. The association between eating and watching movies needs to be broken, which requires that you unlearn that behavior.

Parties, celebrations, and other special occasions like weddings, birthdays, and showers are also social events that cue overeating. If you are asked to bring food to an event, bring something healthy you can snack on, and park your body close to that snack food. Otherwise, use the same strategy as you did for the movies—drink water and eat a small snack before you go to the event. Focus on the conversation and the people who are attending. You can hold a glass of punch or Diet Coke™ in one hand for a long time while you are busy making conversation and interacting with new people.

If you are anxious at social events, practice deep breathing and relaxation techniques (see Appendix E). Don't use food to calm your anxiety. Again, this is a habit you can break.

You may want to look around your workplace. Are there places in that setting that trigger eating? How about the coffee pot? It can be a place of gathering and snacking. We've worked in several offices in which donuts, cake, cookies, and all sorts of goodies are placed by the coffee pot. Naturally, when you go for that cup of java, you are faced with added temptation. You may have to skip the informal chatting in the coffee room and socialize by the water fountain instead.

If a physical space triggers you to eat, change the space. For some of you, this means cleaning out your desks. Hidden in many of those desk drawers are bags of candy and other snack items that you grab when work gets boring or you just need a break.

Grocery shopping can be a tempting activity for overeating, especially if you shop hungry. The best way to avoid this quandary is to eat before you shop, which also helps cut down on buying impulse items. In addition, dietitians frequently recommend that you shop the outside ring of grocery stores where the fresh produce is located. Avoid the cookie aisle and prepackaged foods that are high in trans fat.

Another problem can be cooking. For many of you, cooking means tasting and sampling an entire portion before the food is ever served. You must break that habit while cooking. The smell of food cues you to want to eat, but the extra calories add up. So ask someone else to taste the stew if you think it needs more salt. If you have to stir the pot, do so, but then immediately put down the spoon before you can sample it. And during cleanup, don't eat the leftovers on peoples' plates.

Become comfortable throwing food away in spite of what your mother told you about the starving people in Africa. To our knowledge, no food from your plate has ever been sent to Africa! It's OK. Throw it away! One final word on cooking: Don't cook the things you love that are hard to resist. Your family can survive without your award-winning chocolate cake if having it around trips you up. Remember, you are setting your environment up for success.

As mentioned before, the sight of leftovers can cue the desire to eat, which is why we suggested using foil wrap for foods. When you don't see what the dish is, it isn't as tempting to eat it. Our sight and smell often trigger an urge to overeat. When this happens, we have to decide if we are responding to true physical hunger. For example, whenever I (Dr. Linda) see pies and pastries, I'm ready to eat them whether I'm hungry or not. In part, this is because I grew up with a mother, grandmother, and aunts who all could have been professional pastry chefs. Their desserts are truly out of this world. Just the sight of those desserts brings back great family memories and fun in the kitchen. But if I ate dessert every time I was triggered, I'd weigh a lot more than I do. So when I see a pie sitting on the kitchen counter, I have to ask myself if I'm really hungry or not. Or I have to cut down on my meal in order to enjoy a dessert from time to time. I don't deprive myself, but I also don't indulge every time I see or smell the pastry coming.

Try to think of which social situations or cues trigger you to overeat. Then plan ahead of time how you will handle that situation. Problem solving is actually a useful skill for making life changes because it forces you to anticipate a situation and have a plan. I (Dr. Linda) have worked with several professional chefs who spend their days around food and cooking. Together, we had to plan ways for them to make it through the workday without overeating. First, they wrote down their eating habits while preparing food so we could spot the problem times and items. Then we developed a behavioral plan to ward off overeating. Strategies like keeping a fresh bowl of fruit by their preparation area, drinking lots of water, taking breaks in which they could relax and think, and identifying the type of hunger they experienced (emotional or physical) were all elements of the plan that we implemented.

Increase

Many changes have been suggested—perhaps more than you feel comfortable with. Don't worry. No one expects you to make all the changes at once. In fact, it's a good idea to begin this transformation with a small change. Choose one thing you can do differently for a month and begin by making that change. For example, if you have been a total couch potato, decide to walk five minutes, three times a week. Do that for a month and it will become part of your routine.

Then, add another small change. Perhaps every time you reach to eat out of a need for comfort, you instead choose something from your behavior substitution list (see page 174) and make yourself do that instead. Make that one behavior change your goal for a month. Keep adding changes as you are able. Eventually these small changes will add up. Remember, if you took years to put on the weight, you need to give yourself time to take it off.

Substitute

As you surrender your life to God, another action becomes necessary: forgiveness. Throughout the Word, Jesus is very specific about our need to forgive. "If you forgive men when they sin against you, your heavenly Father will also forgive you" (Matthew 6:14). This is stated as a contingency, meaning we have an active part to accomplish as well as the action of our heavenly Father forgiving us.

Forgiveness, when empowered by God's Spirit, is a process of detaching painful events from our emotional responses to them, thus facilitating the process of healing. When we forgive, we recognize our own failures and are humbled. To forgive and to receive forgiveness are gracious acts of love. These acts have supernatural power to change both the life of the forgiven and the one who forgives. When you look at how God has forgiven you, it moves you to find a way to forgive others even if they have deeply hurt you. Only the cross of Christ makes forgiveness possible.

Forgiveness is inextricably interwoven into Christian salvation. Jesus clearly taught that unless we forgive others, our Heavenly Father cannot forgive us. At first glance, this may appear to be a rigid and rigorous principle, but it is God's means of extending His grace to everyone. When we refuse to forgive, we play "god" in the lives of others and pass our judgment onto them. This interferes with the process of grace Jesus Christ initiated at the cross. Forgiveness means:

· we hand back our rights to God (the rights we usurped from Him) and invite Him to be in charge.
· we obey Jesus' instructions to forgive, and in turn we can be forgiven.
· we no longer energize ourselves with rage or hatred over events or feelings from the past.
· we stop trying to change other people and ask God to do it.

· we begin a process of restitution to right whatever wrongs we may have caused.

Forgiveness can be difficult—almost impossible—for those who have been abused physically, sexually, or even spiritually. It is never easy or instant; it may in fact take years to complete. However, if forgiveness isn't rendered, the injured person remains trapped in the abuse of the past where they endlessly relive the offenses done against them. Our yesterdays must be put in the past so we can fully enjoy today.

The forgiveness process also involves making things right with those we have wounded. This may require us to write letters or phone calls, to repay debts, or to make amends or otherwise do our part in making wrongs as right as possible. This, of course, can result in enormous spiritual blessings, both for others and for ourselves. Sometimes it is difficult to face a person or speak with them on the phone. In such instances, a letter like this one may be the right choice:

Dear Bob,

You may be surprised to be hearing from me, but I have been doing some soul-searching lately. You came to mind and I realized I could have done things differently regarding _____.

I hope you will forgive me. I am making changes in my life so I won't repeat the same mistakes. I hope you are doing well and that God is blessing you.

Sincerely,

It is amazing what a simple letter like that can do to lower the barriers between two people. You will be surprised by the letters you get back and amazed at how ready people are to forgive.

Eliminate

Your goal should be to eat for nourishment and the enjoyment of meals. It's up to you to discover the other functions eating has served in your life. For example, does eating calm you, relax you, numb you, boost your mood, or fill your time? Whatever the function eating has served, you will need to make a change and do something different.

There is an old saying in therapy—if you take something away, replace it with something else or the patient will just substitute another problem-behavior in its place. Many of you can already attest to the truth of this. Perhaps you stopped overeating but began to overspend. Or you stopped overeating and replaced it with another addiction. Obviously, we don't want you to trade addictions or substitute other compulsive behaviors for overeating.

Get at the root of your overeating and resolve it. This may require counseling or additional support to make changes. Don't underestimate the fact that change is difficult. To succeed, we all need the help of family or friends as well as God. Don't be an island determined to do this all alone. Let others come alongside and encourage you. Humble yourself before the Lord and acknowledge your need of Him, and He will lift you up.

Often it is painful to change our behavior. When we have been wronged, it is so much easier to break off all contact and not have a relationship with the person. Yet this isn't what God asks us to do. We must move beyond our hurt and seek forgiveness, as Christ forgave us. If you struggle with this very difficult task, consider this prayer your official starting point:

Dear Lord,

You have commanded me to forgive others, just as You have for-given me through the sacrifice of Your Son, Jesus. I choose to obey, even though this is not easy for me. You listed all of my sins. Then, You nailed them to the cross so that Jesus' blood could pay for them. Help me to release this account to You and not to seek justice for my sake. Help me to trust that You are just and will carry Your will.

Yet, while I transfer this account to You, wounds still remain as a result of this wrong. As I obey You by releasing this person from my debt, I pray You will heal the hurts they have caused me. Help me to trust that You are willing and able to redeem me from the wrongs that have been done against me. If thoughts of revenge recur, I pray You would help me to continually release this person's account to You. Amen.

God sees your heart and knows if you are sincere. He will help you move through the process of forgiveness if you desire to do so. It may help to make a list of those grudges and offenses you have held onto and would like to release. Then, take each item and pray, asking the Lord to forgive you or the person who hurt you.

Releasing these burdens is powerful in the battle to lose weight and keep it off. This is not a step you can skip and still succeed. Take the time, examine your heart, and ask God to show you if there is hidden resentment or judgment. Seek release today.

A Lifelong Journey

If we live our lives without meaning or purpose and become self-obsessed, we've missed what God can do. Don't you want God to take your years of struggle with weight problems and transform it all for His glory? If that is your desire, than you will emerge from this experience stronger and better, and you will be able to help others along the way.

Stay in the race. Press on to the mark. Don't give up. Tarry yet awhile. God's desire is that we all push ourselves to do our best in the race of life. We have to train—read the Word, pray, worship, and develop intimacy with God. Then we develop endurance, the ability to stay in the race no matter how difficult things become. Push yourself in your relationship with Him. Go a little deeper—more faith, more dependence, less of you (physically and emotionally), and more of Him.

Friends, training is hard work, but the payoff feels so good. We are all in training for the eternal. What we do today matters. And we don't have to wait until the race is over to receive rewards. God has set up stations of blessings along the way to encourage us to keep going.

When we train for anything, we must keep our minds fixed on the goal. Know where you are heading and keep your mind fixed on getting there. Will you endure the hardships around you? Will you be faithful to the end? Can God count on you? Or will you give up and complain that life is just too hard? We pray you stay in the race no matter how difficult it becomes.

Father,

For everyone who feels like giving up, for everyone who thinks they can't go on, give them a revelation of Your love and help. You desire them to go the distance. Your reward is great, both today and eternally. Help us to keep our eyes fixed on You and the final prize. Give us the strength to endure when we think we can't. More than anything, give us Your presence. Connect us with those who will encourage and share in the race with us until the end—and may we be strengthened through the love of Jesus Christ. Amen.

10

Community—the Connection Cornerstone

American Christianity is influenced by the culture in which it operates. We live in a society known for placing value on independence, self-sufficiency, and what is called "rugged individualism." Historically, autonomy, individual drive, and self-motivation have been admired characteristics, yet this is not the biblical practice suggested for the body of Christ.

Relationship is characteristic of the Godhead—they are three in one. The Trinity enjoys fellowship. Relationship has existed from the beginning of time. Since the beginning of creation, God knew it was good for a man to have a helper, which is why He created woman.

While God's triune relationship is often mysterious to our human understanding, we do know that God so loved the world that He sent His only Son Jesus to die and take the sins of the world for our redemption. Out of love, God found a way to relate to us through His Son. While on earth, Jesus was highly relational as He communed with His Father, chose disciples, spent time with sinners, and even gave of His time to play with children.

A central message of Jesus' teaching was for us to live in unity with one another. When Jesus returned to the Father, the Holy Spirit was sent as Comforter. If we explore the beginnings of church history in the book of Acts, we find a record of how Christianity was practiced under the power of the Holy Spirit. As the church developed and spread, believers learned to live together, sharing freely with one another while maintaining meaningful fellowship. Even in the face of strong personalities and differences, the church found a way to listen and to submit to one another in Christian love. Because of the dedication of this early church in fasting and in prayer, people were released to do incredible miracles and extraordinary acts. Through the power of the Holy Spirit and the unity and love practiced in community, believers were healed. Now delivered, we must resist spiritual oppression. In Christian community, we learn to love, heal, and live together as one body.

Lose It For Life believes strongly in the connections made in Christian community. We need each other. As we encourage one another and lift each other up in prayer, we move forward in the Christian life in ways not possible as a lone sojourner. Relationships are important in order to meet our needs for intimacy and support, but also to grow and avoid relapse.

RISE to the Challenge

In order to RISE above the challenges, we need connection and community. Add these goals to your program:

REDUCE: negative relationships that sabotage your program.

INCREASE: connection with others, social skills, and community.

SUBSTITUTE: the healing of community and connection for the belief that you must go it alone.

ELIMINATE: the lone ranger mentality and toxic relationships that undermine your success.

Fight Disconnection

When we are obsessed with food and weight, we often hide while feeling outcast and alienated from others. Embarrassed by what we weigh and feeling out of control, many of us feel like second-class citizens and pull back from active involvement with others. Instead of being our true selves, we do things to please others and hope they never see who we really are for fear they won't like us. Maybe you've been bullied or rejected because of your weight. Consequently, you've pulled back from others in fear of more of the same. People who grow up in overly critical homes or homes in which they were teased about their weight often try to hide within social situations rather than connect.

Food obsessions involve time and energy that take you away from other activities. When you are overweight, you leave early, come late, sit by yourself, and refuse to share certain parts of yourself with others. There is an assumption that once the weight is gone, you'll become a social butterfly. However, Cathy found out that "flying solo" wasn't a good idea.

March 15, 2004—I wish I could say that after losing 119 pounds all my food issues are finally behind me. I guess somewhere in my imagination I believed that if I ever lost this much weight again I would surely be floating from social event to social event never desiring to eat junk food or binge again. It was going to be great! I guess this is a good time for a reality check! I was so wrong.

The truth is that some days now are just as hard as the first day I began this journey. There are days I make poor choices and fall off the wagon and, as crazy as it sounds, there are days I am tempted to go back to my old habits. Changing patterns and habits is hard. Maturing and dying to self is hard.

But letting go of God's hand is detrimental. I've noticed that just when I think I have this whole food addiction thing licked—and I start flying solo—I tend to crash. But the Lord has been so faithful. He knows my heart. As I cry out to Him to help me change, He always provides a way of escape for me. How wonderful to have a Daddy that loves me this much.

I am beginning to understand that this will never be an easy feat. Good health—emotional, spiritual, and physical—does not just happen. It is truly a gift from God. We must do our part and allow Him to do His part. It's a journey taken one day at a time.

—CATHY

When someone loses as much weight as Cathy did, one of the most common expectations is that life will be dramatically different. This is particularly true from a social perspective. There are assumptions that when the weight is gone, the dates will be many and the whole outlook will be different, including being able to socially engage for the first time. It will be magical, or so the person thinks!

Then the weight comes off and reality hits. *Where are all those new party invitations? Why isn't that healthy, trim woman (ME!) getting invited out?* The disappointment is that all this effort has not resulted in a new and exciting social life. Why? Because losing weight doesn't necessarily change who you are inside!

When you spend your life as an overweight person, you learn to feel uneasy in social situations and avoid and withdraw. There is work to be done on the inside of the person too—to build confidence and be put in new social situations. This means taking new risks, which is never easy. A person can still struggle with major insecurities even when their body looks healthier. So part of the work of losing it for life is to venture into the uncertain and unpredictable world of people and relationships.

You Need the Body

It helps to remember the source of your true worth. Jesus Christ says you are already accepted, loved, and special. Other people may not always be so positive and affirming. However, there are those people who will be, and you must find them and make a connection. You need their support and encouragement.

One reason people struggle even when they know their relationship with Christ is vital to success is because they are not connected to a community of fellow believers. No matter how successful you are at doing this program, you need connections with people who can help when you feel down or want to give in and give up. As one woman who was losing weight confided,

> *People are always asking me for advice. I don't want to give advice! I'm still dealing with weight loss myself. Yes, I've had some success, but I'm still working on issues and prefer to talk to those who are struggling. I don't want to "help" everyone else in the way I used to. That was my old pattern and it took me away from doing what I needed to do to help myself. I think I can most help by being honest and saying this isn't easy, but that one day at a time, I'm making it.*

When you are the consummate giver and never expect to receive in a relationship, you tend to attract needy people who can suck you dry. And then, guess what? You feel empty and use food to fill that void again. This woman knew she needed others to help her and wasn't in a position to be their expert. Community is so important in this journey because it links you with support and encouragement for these moments of difficulty. In the body of Christ, when you feel strong, you encourage another. When you are down, another person encourages you. This give-and-take is the basis for healthy relationships.

Revisit Social Skills

When you begin to take risks socially, you must also take a hard look at your social skills. Maybe you need to be more assertive, learn how to initiate conversation, or demonstrate a new interest in others. Weight loss will boost your confidence, but it won't teach you social skills.

If you've spent a lifetime hiding and you come out of the eating closet, you may have to practice new skills. So today, make it your goal to approach someone you would like to get to know better. Find out an interest he or she has and begin to ask about it. Broaden your own interests now that you aren't so obsessed with food and eating. Try a new activity and see how it feels. Certainly it will feel a little scary at first. That's OK. It gets easier the more you do it. If you aren't invited to the party, bring the party to you! That's right. You throw a party and ask people to come. If you are tired of no social life, create one. Start small. Ask a few old friends to come and include one or two new ones. Don't make the focus of the party food or drink (time to let go of that crutch). Instead, have a structured activity like playing Trivial Pursuit™. Then relax, laugh, and enjoy the fun. The more you practice doing things that are uncomfortable, the easier they will become.

Don't Alienate Yourself

Overeating can keep us from the very people we need support from. In addition to shame, fear, and embarrassment, or thinking we lack good social skills, we can stay isolated because of pride. We convince ourselves that needing others is too painful or is weakness. We really don't need people to help us in life because we've bought the American idealism of doing it on our own. We have to gut it out and our failure to do so is because we lack willpower, not because we need others along the way.

In some cases, our lack of experience with healthy relationships keeps us from trying. Growing up alone and isolated, we see no benefit in relationships. Our experience only brought hurt. Or in cases where relationship may have started out strong, we were betrayed or disappointed. People cannot be trusted. In the end, you believe you will be rejected.

Many of us just give up on relationships and fail to make the distinction between the benefits of healthy relationships and the needy and overly dependent relationships in which we may be entwined. The former are healthy; the latter are toxic. Because we fail to define who we are outside of our weight, we lack appropriate boundaries within our relationships and self-care. We want people to fill those empty places, even when we know this isn't healthy. So we pull away altogether, deciding we are too needy and too messed up for this relationship.

Yet even with all our reasons for pulling back and protecting ourselves from hurt or pain, we still desire connection. We were created to relate to God and others. It is in relationships that we grow and learn about ourselves. Through our experiences with others, we define how we think and feel. Attachment is a basic need that never goes away but longs to be met. And while we try to meet that need through eating, the need is never satisfied.

The need for connection is not unhealthy, but how you meet that need can be. In God's kingdom, nobody is more important than the next. You aren't less because you weigh more. We approach each other with humility and must have the courage to be open to what we can receive from others. Yes, we can be rejected, but we can also find people who will accept and love us no matter what we weigh or how many times we fail. If we don't allow bad relationships to derail our efforts, we can have meaningful connections and our needs will be met.

Healthy relationships include loving God, ourselves, and others. We don't love with a puffed up sense of importance. We love because God loves us and has purpose and meaning for our lives. As we surrender to that purpose and plan, we purposefully connect with others to accomplish what we can't accomplish alone. Connection brings healing and healing brings joy.

When we are willing to be open, transparent, and vulnerable to others, we break free of the isolation that keeps us hidden in the dark. We feel God's love because we aren't moving in pretense. We learn to accept who we are because we are in process. We ask for healing so we can grow and give to others and find rest.

Food, Marriage, and Fidelity

In some marriages, weight creates a sense of protection. We referred early on to the idea that being heavy can protect you from your own sexual impulses or the impulses of others.[68] People who aren't sure they can resist sexual temptations may stay heavy as a way to control their impulsivity. Also, the fear of feeling sexually attractive makes some people uncomfortable, in part because they aren't certain they can control their impulses.

How many times have you or someone you know complained that the necessary support for weight loss was lacking? Those around us and in our intimate relationships can actually sabotage our efforts. For example, the best way to prevent your spouse from losing weight is to demand that he or she do so. After years of working with couples, this fact is certain: When a spouse demands weight loss, weight loss undergoes a death sentence. Why? Because there is something about a demand that says you don't accept the partner as he or she is. Acceptance is instead conditioned on the basis of weight. A demand to look different is often accompanied by criticism and comparisons which usually signal deeper issues in a relationship that must be addressed.

Another interesting observation is the number of husbands who seem to sabotage their wives' efforts to lose weight. In some cases, husbands worry that their wives' thinner appearances will make them more vulnerable to other men. Alternatively, if one spouse takes responsibility for a weight problem, there may be the expectation that the other spouse will tackle a specific problem like anger, drinking, or gambling. We have also seen cases of sabotage because spouses are unwilling to have their routines and eating habits altered for the sake of their partner's healthy desire to lose weight.

I (Dr. Linda) remember one woman I worked with whose husband brought home candy almost every day despite the fact that she was paying me to help her lose weight. Repeatedly, she asked him to stop bringing candy into the house. Yet he never stopped. At my request, he came to a counseling session. I discovered that he was worried that he would be asked to make changes in his own life if his wife overcame her weight problem. And while he didn't like the fact that his wife was significantly overweight, he preferred to keep life the way it was—with the pressure off. He later admitted that he felt inadequate to make changes in his own life and secretly did not want his wife to succeed because he would feel more like a failure.

Weight loss efforts can also be sabotaged because you've spent your entire life playing the victim. While this isn't a role you probably desire, it may be a familiar one. To move out of the victim position would mean forgiving people and making other changes. Giving up anything you know well to move into the unknown is always a bit unsettling, but the gains are certainly worth a bit of anxiety. A lack of trust is at the root of this problem. You must trust that being obedient to God's Word, as well as forgiving others' wrongs and extending grace, will turn out beneficial to you and others in the long run. As we discussed in the last chapter, don't allow bitterness to prevent you from moving forward.

Spousal support and the support of families and intimate others is very important when it comes to losing weight.[69] Talk about your goals with loved ones before you begin any program. Discuss whether there are hidden fears or relationship concerns about your losing weight. Then work together as much as possible. The best situation is when your intimate relationships can be part of your support system.

Embrace Community

If you decide to be more vulnerable and open your life up to others, recognize that it won't be easy or a positive experience 100 percent of the time. You'll have times of frustration and you'll learn who can handle your openness and who cannot. There are people who are not trustworthy, and you must be discerning about who you will open up to. Yet be careful how you do this! Paul addresses how we are to behave with one another in Romans 14:1-9:

Welcome with open arms fellow believers who don't see things the way you do. And don't jump all over them every time they do or say something you don't agree with—even when it seems that they are strong on opinions but weak in the faith department. Remember, they have their own history to deal with. Treat them gently.

For instance, a person who has been around for a while might well be convinced that he can eat anything on the table, while another, with a different background, might assume all Christians should be vegetarians and eat accordingly. But since both are guests at Christ's table, wouldn't it be terribly rude if they fell to criticizing what the other ate or didn't eat? God, after all, invited them both to the table. Do you have any business crossing people off the guest list or interfering with God's welcome? If there are corrections to be made or manners to be learned, God can handle that without your help.

Or, say, one person thinks that some days should be set aside as holy and another thinks that each day is pretty much like any other. There are good reasons either way. So, each person is free to follow the convictions of conscience.

What's important in all this is that if you keep a holy day, keep it for God's sake; if you eat meat, eat it to the glory of God and thank God for prime rib; if you're a vegetarian, eat vegetables to the glory of God and thank God for broccoli. None of us are permitted to insist on our own way in these matters. It's God we are answerable to—all the way from life to death and everything in between—not each other. That's why Jesus lived and died and then lived again: so that he could be our Master across the entire range of life and death, and free us from the petty tyrannies of each other. (MSG)

If we allow Jesus to be our Master who can "free us from the petty tyrannies of each other," dynamic things will happen. We all have differences that can divide us if we let them. However, we are called to unity and we should work out our differences in Christian love and maturity. The unity that results will create an atmosphere for healing. Make it your goal to find people who you can trust and be authentic with, who will maintain confidences and pray with you. Work on your differences with others and learn to live in Christian love.

Relationships are work because they often act as mirrors to our problems. In intimacy, we see our weaknesses and need for God's help. As we grow, we become aware of our separateness, but also our need for each other. As we learn to define who we are, set boundaries, deal with conflict, and manage differences, we grow if we stay connected to others in the process.

What should we look for when it comes to building relationships with one another? Ephesians 4:2 says, "Be completely humble and gentle; be patient, bearing with one another in love." We are to pursue community with one another and be patient and humble in the process.

Jesus recognized the need for community in His darkest hour. He took His disciples with Him to pray as He faced the biggest challenge of His earthly life—the cross. As He hung on the cross, He thought of others and even welcomed a thief into Paradise! He also arranged for John, the beloved, to care for His mother. And in those last moments before His death, He cried out from a sense of estrangement, "My God, my God, why have you forsaken me?" (Matthew 27:46). For a brief moment, He felt abandoned by the Father and became a curse for us, as Paul reminds us in Galatians.

Jesus is all about community. He tells us that people will know us by our love (John 13:35) and that we are to love one another. When you face any difficult change or trial in your life, support and community make the difference in your ability to survive and come through the trial. Seek wise counsel from those who can help you. Be responsive to your pastors and leaders who will provide spiritual accountability. Take advantage of counselors and therapists who can help you sort out the complexity of weight loss as it applies to you and your specific life. Be persistent and have the courage to be open in relationships with others.

As you seek a more intimate connection with God through your church, you may find that you redefine your weight problem as a fruit problem. Fruit is the visible part of our lives that others can see. Galatians 5:22-23 (AMP) describes what builds healthy relationships in our lives: "But the fruit of the [Holy] Spirit [the work which His presence within accomplishes] is love, joy (gladness), peace, patience (an even temper, forbearance), kindness, goodness (benevolence), faithfulness, gentleness (meekness, humility), self-control (self-restraint, continence). Against such things there is no law [that can bring a charge]."

Do you evidence the fruit of the Spirit is in you when it comes to dealing with other people? As you submit yourself to God's growing and pruning process, ask Him to put you with others who are committed to bearing this type of fruit also. Healthy communities bear this kind of fruit. Look for it.

All praise to the God and Father of our Master, Jesus the Messiah! Father of all mercy! God of all healing counsel! He comes alongside us when we go through hard times, and before you know it, he brings us alongside someone else who is going through hard times so that we can be there for that person just as God was there for us. —2 CORINTHIANS 1:3-4 (MSG)

What a fabulous verse! God comes alongside of us when we go through difficulty. That in and of itself is reassuring, but there is even more—God will use us to help someone else who is going through a hard time as well. In God's economy, nothing is ever wasted, not even pain!

We can never know God's plans or His gain from our loss, unless we give Him our misery and allow Him to transform it into a mission for our lives. Once our loss and pain point us to God's grace, we can also lead others into His grace. In doing so, we partner with God as He accomplishes His purposes. After we emerge from our own despair, become transparent, and candidly share our victories, we will be in a position to share our struggles and God's power to overcome, attracting others into His grace.

God's church is our earthly home. Embrace the love and support He has instituted for you and build on that connection for life.

11
Pressing On—Keeping It Off

Grant me the serenity to accept things
I cannot change, the courage to change
the things I can, and the wisdom
to know the difference. Amen.

By now you know that losing it for life is not something you do quickly. Rather, you are engaged in an ongoing transformation that comes through connection and community and practicing what you know works: exercising and eating healthily. It is possible to lose weight and keep it off. However, the journey required to make necessary changes isn't easy and doesn't end with losing the amount of weight desired.

We can know what to do, do it, and still slip back into old patterns of behavior, thinking, and feeling. In fact, John 6:66 reminds us that we can know the truth and still turn from it. Whenever you deal with a chronic problem like weight loss and maintenance, you have to be willing to do whatever it takes to avoid relapse. Planning is key to preventing relapse. You have to begin recovery and follow through or you place yourself at risk for relapse.

Relapse is more than a "slip" or return to overeating. An overeating episode is preceded by a process—one that generally involves a predictable progression that gradually moves you farther and farther away from doing what you know worked in the first place until, ultimately, you lose control. You revert to old patterns. For example, your thoughts focus on failure; your feelings on disgust and self-hate; and your actions on giving up or responding to unhealthy guilt in an unhealthy manner. All of these instances will bring you back to feeling failed and hopeless.

Yet if you can recognize the signs of relapse early, you will know when you are entering dangerous waters and choose to get back on track. If you can assess your situation and be watchful of the warning signs, you can avoid relapse.

The Signs of Relapse

1. DISHONESTY
   Feeling: You feel victimized and entitled.
   Thinking: You're not at fault; the reasons for overeating are rational.
   Action: You lie and present a false self once again hidden under the protection of fat.

2. NEGATIVE SELF-CENTEREDNESS AND PITY
   Feeling: You feel sorry for yourself; you revert to the victim position.
   Thinking: You feel the world is against you, owes you, and revolves around you; resentful, defensive, and overly sensitive.
   Action: You can do anything you want to do because nothing is helpful.

3. LOW FRUSTRATION TOLERANCE
   Feeling: You feel irritation, excitement, impatience, dissatisfaction.
   Thinking: You need it now. People aren't acting right. This is taking too much time.
   Action: You experience impulsivity and arguments.

4. ANXIETY

Feeling: You feel pressured and worried; strained, a lack of confidence, and free-floating fear.

Thinking: You are confused and indecisive.

Action: You are paralyzed; no plan to follow.

5. GRANDIOSITY

Feeling: You feel overconfident, powerful, and arrogant.

Thinking: You're the exception to the rule. You've got it made. You'll show them. You need to be the center of attention.

Action: You play counselor with others, impress others with accomplishments, need to have the best; martyrdom; generous to a fault.

6. PERFECTIONISM

Feeling: You feel guilt over never doing enough; constantly driven to do more.

Thinking: Nothing is ever correct. You must make up for past mistakes.

Action: You are cut off from others.

7. THERE-AND-THEN LIVING (opposite of here-and-now living)

Feeling: You feel fear of the future, regret of the past, resentment.

Thinking: You experience wishful thinking, fantasy; "If only . . ."

Action: You live according to "shoulds" rather than needs; needs not met in the present.

8. DEFIANCE

Feeling: You feel inner conflict.

Thinking: No one knows but you.

Action: You run from help and experience destructive expression of feelings, open rebellion.

9. ISOLATION

Feeling: You feel boredom, loneliness; "I don't belong."

Thinking: You don't need anyone. You can do it yourself. No one cares.

Action: You experience withdrawal, reject help.

The Phases of Relapse

Because relapse is not just one episode of overeating but a gradual process that builds over time, you should also be aware of the phases of relapse. If you note similarities between yourself and any of these descriptions, make immediate changes to compensate.

Complacency

Complacency is the first phase of relapse and begins when you stop doing what you know helps. This can happen because you get bored with your plan, drop your plan, become tired of making changes, feel upset or overwhelmed with all the changes required, or begin to believe you don't have the same needs that led you to surrender in the first place.

Giving up weight and food obsession involves moving into unfamiliar territory where weight no longer protects you from attention, intimacy, and vulnerability. It can also mean creating instant space from others, relieving sexual tension, and providing new excuses. While you can intellectually know these are all good things to give up, you have to be willing to stay the course when these issues are confronted.

You may stop going to counseling or support groups or activities that keep you connected and accountable to others and begin to think you don't need any more help. Or you may become too involved with others and not set appropriate boundaries. As a result, you can become lost in the needs of others and lose sight of your own.

Negative thinking can take hold in which you deny negative emotions such as fear and live in a fantasy world. There you daydream, set unrealistic expectations, intellectualize, engage in naval gazing, become easily angered and dissatisfied, and begin to obsess about food and weight as you entertain wishful thoughts and stop doing what has led you to lose the weight in the first place.

Confusion

Next, confusion sets in. You begin to doubt that anything works or will make a difference. You become double-minded. The issues related to losing weight and the lifestyle changes needed are doubted as you settle back into thinking you don't need to do all that is required. Perhaps your weight problems weren't that problematic and all this change isn't necessary. Doubt is the main thought—doubt about the depths of your difficulties or the need for recovery, help, or ongoing support.

You find yourself disconnecting from your support system and from people to whom you have been accountable. Self-doubt and low self-esteem occupy your thoughts. More expectations turn in to "false hopes." Problem solving becomes difficult and you give in to living for the moment. Your plan goes by the wayside. This leads to irrational and inconsistent behavior.

Compromise

As complacency and confusion grow, you begin to engage in behaviors that set you up for problems once again. Overeating creeps back in and you rationalize, "It was only this one time. I'll be OK." And you return to old patterns of thinking and acting, using food to comfort and to fill emotional needs once again. Food, weight, and eating occupy your day as you think about the next meal or what you will eat in the next hour. You give in to impulsive eating, seeking momentary relief from this new life stress. The weight gain starts to creep back up.

Thoughts of apprehension and "If only" statements fill your head. Giving in to the moment leads to an attitude of not caring when it comes to food and eating. You give up your routine with exercise and meal planning, rationalizing that action in spite of your obvious need.

Your emotional states intensify, especially anger and dissatisfaction, because you are not dealing with life head-on and are instead allowing negativity, blame, dishonesty, and other destructive emotions to grow.

Because you are unwilling to confront the issues related to overeating and refuse to take responsibility, you further separate yourself from your support system and those who will lovingly hold you accountable. You are back to thinking your own effort and self-will will prevail when you decide to get serious again.

Catastrophe

Any feeling of control over the food is gone and you are bingeing, overeating, and overindulging once again. And since you have "blown it," why care? There are no attempts to limit what you eat, when, and how much. Sedentary once again, you feel physically sluggish, emotionally drained and overwhelmed, depressed, anxious, and disconnected from others. Thus, you engage in more risk and irresponsible behavior with food and your eating. The main feeling at this stage is helplessness and hopelessness. You are in trouble and have gained a significant amount of weight back, and there is no end in sight to that state of being.

Protection from Relapse

In order to prevent relapse, you want to establish a system of protection. This system should include the following components:

An Exercise Plan

Exercise isn't something you do to lose weight and then quit; it promotes health, enhances your sense of well-being, and is a form of stress reduction. It is a natural form of stimulating the body and also providing relaxation. When you exercise, you feel you've accomplished something. We recommend trying to involve your entire family in exercise as a way to make it easier to do. For example, learn a new sport together, go on after-dinner walks, or take up a new hobby like dancing or hiking. Exercise and physical activity are essential to a healthy lifestyle and must be a part of your regular, daily routine.

Nutrition

Changes in your eating habits must also become habit in order to prevent relapse. Remember to eat foods high in protein and low in sugar in order to rebuild tissue and stabilize your blood sugar and moods. Reduce your fat intake, especially trans fats. Keep your eating habits healthy by only eating at the table, eating smaller, more frequent meals during the day, and eliminating high-sugar sodas and caffeine. These changes are about living a healthy lifestyle—not just dieting and losing weight. Make good nutrition a lifelong change.

Rest and Relaxation

Both must be scheduled. Take scheduled time-outs and regularly practice relaxation methods such as deep breathing and deep muscle relaxation. Work on keeping your body de-stressed. Stress leads to overeating for so many people. Work hard but learn to play and rest as well.

Think Lifestyle

The overall goal of making changes is to have them become part of your lifestyle. Everything you've learned and are applying to your life will become part of who you are and a lasting change. Losing weight for life is about thinking with a long-term perspective and making choices that will give your body good health.

Keep Growing

We must continue to grow and mature as we make it our goal to imitate Christ in all we do. You may need counseling and support groups to help move you forward in this area. Interaction with the church community provides numerous opportunities to grow: Cell groups, prayer groups, seminars, classes, and other activities are opportunities for you to spiritually grow and mature. Take advantage of all the materials and planned meetings designed to help you develop a deeper walk with God.

Spiritual maturity does not come about in isolation. Becoming part of a church community is essential to your growth as a person. As we interact with others, we have numerous opportunities to practice being like Christ and loving one another. In addition, others can mentor us in Christian maturity and help keep us accountable.

Living One Day at a Time

The changes you are making and the personal growth and maturity that come with accepting responsibility for your health and well-being are best lived out one day at a time. It's easy to become overwhelmed, stressed, and discontent, so stay focused on today. Ask God to give you the grace you need to meet the challenges each day presents.

Avoid thinking in an "If only . . ." fashion; it is not compatible with surrender and reflects an attitude of discontent while also being a form of fantasy thinking. Look to the past to learn from your mistakes, but don't stay there in unhealthy guilt! There is forgiveness for what is confessed and past. Remember that how you live today sets your course for the future, so live well!

Accept Accountability

In order to be accountable, you cannot hide from the truth. Confess your sins and do not hide from hidden abuses or fantasies. All of us need spiritual support and thus need to find those who can support us in prayer, give and receive comfort, and share encouragement. You can benefit greatly from the experience of others. Stay teachable and keep a humble spirit. Accept advice and learn to listen. Take seriously Proverbs 15:22: "Plans fail for lack of counsel, but with many advisors they succeed."

Rely on God

Though it may sound like a cliché, God does have a plan and purpose for your life. He doesn't necessarily reveal those plans moment by moment, but God wants us to trust Him and take Him at His word. Nothing is too hard for God. "Jesus looked at them and said, 'With man this is impossible, but not with God; all things are possible with God'" (Mark 10:27). What an incredible statement from God's mouth!

Now believe it and act on its truth. Even though we know God is never late or early, waiting for His perfect timing requires patience and faith. He sees the big picture and intimate details of your life. His plans for you are good, but you must trust in His promises.

Spiritual Disciplines

It is absolutely essential to your spiritual growth and health to practice the spiritual disciplines of prayer, worship, confession, Bible study, giving, fasting, submission, service, and forgiving. Scripture is our one reliable source of truth and instructs us on the life that will bring satisfaction and victory. Intercession and confession bring us into communion with our Father. Praise and worship take us into the presence of God. In His presence there is joy and healing. We live in a time of great spiritual warfare, one in which the enemy of our souls will contest our spiritual progress at every turn. We must live godly lives and develop as God has instructed according to His will.

Protect the Spiritual Gains Made

The Christian gospel brings a profound message about earthly evil being transformed into eternal good: weakness into strength, tragedy into triumph, loss into gain, mortality into immortality, death into life. These concepts might be superficially discounted as theological abstractions, except that they translate into inescapable, day-by-day "miracles" that are clearly evident in the lives of Christian believers throughout the world.

The cosmic turning point in the transformation of evil-to-good is the death and resurrection of Jesus Christ. We activate this process in our lives through faith in God's Son, through hope in His good and loving character, and through relinquishment of our lives to His flawless will.

The process of surrendering to God's love and authority is a lifelong process. By the time we have made our way through the process of spiritual transformation, we know we need other Christians to help us stay on the right path. Without them, we are likely to return to patterns of secrecy, sin, and sickness. Yet when we place ourselves in a position of accountability to others, we invite their scrutiny.

At first this goes against our natural bent and seems like an invasion of our privacy, but accountability to others is an invaluable means of preventing a recurrence of sinful behavior. The removal of "secrets" from our lives was essential to our healing; now we need to introduce spiritual disciplines in our lives so that we are not entrapped by either overconfidence or a return to secret sins.

Paul wrote, "We should be decent and true in everything we do, so that everyone can approve of our behavior . . . let the Lord Jesus Christ take control of you, and don't think of ways to indulge your evil desires"

(Romans 13:13-14 NLT). We are able to remain "decent and true" only because God is with us, upholding us, and giving us new life. By continually surrendering to His will and through ongoing and honest accountability to trustworthy individuals, we are transformed. Yet we must never forget where we came from and how we got where we are, just as 2 Peter 1:5-9 urges us:

> So don't lose a minute in building on what you've been given, complementing your basic faith with good character, spiritual understanding, alert discipline, passionate patience, reverent wonder, warm friendliness, and generous love, each dimension fitting into and developing the others. With these qualities active and growing in your lives, no grass will grow under your feet; no day will pass without its reward as you mature in your experience of our Master Jesus. Without these qualities you can't see what's right before you, oblivious that your old sinful life has been wiped off the books. (MSG)

Scripture indicates that human willfulness is at odds with God's plan for His people. He created us to be entirely dependent upon Him. We must continue to repent of our sins and to return to His ways. He wants us to communicate with Him in prayer. He also has indicated in His description of the multidimensional body of Christ (1 Corinthians 12; Romans 12) that we are meant to be dependent on other Christians. Our sinful nature will always tell us that we can handle life quite well on our own. However, God's Word and painful experiences remind us that we can't. Preservation is a key to spiritual renewal and transformation which means we:

· establish boundaries to prevent a return to sick, sinful behaviors.
· continue to forgive and be forgiven, including ourselves when we slip.

- remain accountable to others and keep their confidences in turn.
- choose to be part of a godly community.
- practice the spiritual disciplines on a daily basis.
- develop with God's help a deep and godly character.
- continue the process of surrender—day by day, year by year.

Friends, there is reason to be hopeful about this journey. While we all struggle with difficulty and pain, we can learn to surrender our all to God. He wants us to succeed in this journey, because to do so means to find freedom in Christ and a release from the bondage of overeating. But only with God's leading can you lose it for life and stay on this journey. To Him be the glory!

A Personal Note from
Steve Arterburn

God loves you as you are—please know and believe this truth. But He also wants you to find the weight that is right for you and maintain that weight. Truly, everything and anything is possible for your future. If you surrender your life to God, humble yourself to get the assistance you need, and willingly make the changes you need to make, you will lose the weight and be free of it for life.

Don't be discouraged. If you struggle, and wonder why, understand that the journey is difficult! All of us who struggle with overeating share your pain. The reality is that you can stumble back and you can stumble forward . . . just don't ever give up. Thousands of people have successfully traveled this road. This can be your story, too, but you must do whatever it takes to win this battle.

God is for you. Dr. Linda and I are for you. The healing community at loseitforlife.com is for you. So come, begin this journey, and look toward the freedom we have experienced that can also be yours. And if I can help you in any way, e-mail me: Sarterburn@newlife.com.

Steve

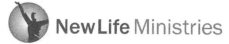

NewLife Ministries

If you are interested in attending a Lose It For Life Institute, call 1-800-NEWLIFE or visit our web sites at NewLife.com or LoseItForLife.com.

ENDNOTES

1   Hellmich, Nanci. "Obesity in America Is Worse Than Ever," *USA Today.* October 9, 2002.

2   Mayo Clinic Women's Health Source. *Causes of Obesity,* Vol. 6, No. 4. April 2002.

3   Ibid.

4   Hellmich, Nanci. "Obesity in America Is Worse Than Ever," *USA Today.* October 9, 2002.

5   Crowther, J.H., Wolf, E.M., & Sherwood, N. "Epidemiology of Bulimia Nervosa," in M. Crowther, D.L. Tennenbaum. S.E. Hobfoll, & M.A.P. Stephens (Eds.), *The Etiology of Bulimia Nervosa: The Individual and Familial Context* (pp. 1-26). Washington, D.C.: Taylor & Francis. 1992.

6   Arterburn, S. & Stoop, D. *Seven Keys to Spiritual Renewal.* Wheaton, IL: Tyndale House Publishers, 1998.

7   Parker-Pope, Tara. "The Diet That Works: What Science Tells Us About Weight Loss," *Wall Street Journal.* April 22, 2003.

8   Ibid.

9   Adapted from Virtue, Doreen. *Constant Craving A-Z.* Carlsbad, CA: Hay House, 1999. Retrieved online May 10, 2004, from http://www.utexas.edu/student/cmhc/outreach/8traits.html.

10 Mayo Clinic Women's Health Source. *Causes of Obesity,* Vol. 6, No. 4. April 2002.

11 Retrieved online May 11, 2004, from http://instruct1.cit.cornell.edu/courses/ns421/BMR.html.

12 Ibid.

13 Hoffman, J. Scientific American.com. "Ask the Experts: Biology. Why Does Fat Deposit on the Thighs and Hips of Women and Around the Stomachs of Men?" Retrieved online May 23, 2004. <_question.cfm?articleID=000D5A77 FA90-1D89-B3B9809EC588EEDF&pageNumber=2&cat ID=3.

14 Ibid.

15 Mann, Denise. "Stress May Cause Fat Around the Midsection in Lean Women." September 22, 2000. Retrieved May 23, 2004, online at http://my.webmd.com/content/article/28/1728_ 61643.htm?lastselectedguid={5FE84E90-BC77-4056-A91C-9531713CA348}.

16 Bowman, Lee. "Sleep Loss a Factor in Holiday Weight Gain," *The Orange County Register.* December 25, 2002.

17 Su, MD, Robert K. Posted in the Virginia Pain Clinic, Portsmouth Virginia. Used with permission. 1985.

18 http://www.niddk.nih.gov/health/nutrit/pubs/health.htm#diabetes. Retrieved April 29, 2004.

19 http://www.niddk.nih.gov/health/nutrit/pubs/health.htm#heartdisease. Retrieved April 29, 2004.

20 Ibid.

21 Ibid.

22 Taken from http://www.niddk.nih.gov/health/nutrit/pubs/health.htm#sleep. Retrieved April 29, 2004.

23 Taken from http://www.niddk.nih.gov/health/nutrit/pubs/health.htm#arthritis. Retrieved April 29, 2004.

24 Taken from http://www.niddk.nih.gov/health/nutrit/pubs/health.htm#gallbladder. Retrieved April 29, 2004.

25 Taken from http://www.niddk.nih.gov/health/nutrit/pubs/health.htm#liver. Retrieved April 29, 2004.

26 From the Metropolitan Life Insurance Company. See www.halls.md/ideal-weight/met.htm for the pros and cons of these charts.

27 Stedman, Nancy. "The Hunger-proof Diet." *Reader's Digest,* p. 96. January 1999.

28 Platkin, Charles. "If You Want to Lose Weight, You Need More than a Miracle Food," *The Honolulu Advisor.* Shape Up. November 27, 2002.

29 Davis, Lisa. "Holy Cow, Look What Makes You Thin," *Reader's Digest,* pp. 107-111. July 2002.

30 "'Oreos Too Dangerous for Our Kids,' Suit Says" *The Orange County Register.* May 13, 2003.

31 Heller, Samantha. "The Hidden Killer." *Men's Health,* pp. 116-118. September 2003.

32 Kluger, Jeffrey. "Fessing Up to Fats," *Time.* July 21, 2003.

33 "The Hidden Killer." *Men's Health,* pp. 116-118. September 2003.

34 *The Society for Neuroscience.* "Brain Briefings: Sugar Addiction." October 2003. Retrieved online from http://web.sfn.org/content/Publications/BrainBriefings/sugar.html.

35 Sorgen, Carol. "Snack Attack: Coping with Cravings." October 14, 2002. Retrieved online May 26, 2004, from http://my.webmd.com/content/article/51/40783.htm?z=2731_00000_0000 _ep_01.

36 Engler, M.B. *Journal of the American College of Nutrition,* Vol. 23: pp. 197-204. News release, University of California, San Francisco. June 2004.

37 Stone, Felicity. "Health Tip: Breakfast Benefits." Forbes.com Retrieved online May 27, 2004, from http://www.forbes.com/health/feeds/hscout/2004/05/20/hscout518894.html.

38 Parker-Pope, Tara. "The Diet that Works: What Science Tells Us About Weight Loss," *Wall Street Journal*. April 22, 2003.

39 Hellmich, Nanci. "'Clean Your Plate' Tradition Coming Back to Bite Us." *USA Today*. September 24, 2003.

40 *Men's Health*, Nutritional Briefs, p. 50. May 2003.

41 Parker-Pope, Tara. "The Diet that Works: What Science Tells Us About Weight Loss," *Wall Street Journal*. April 22, 2003.

42 Wansink, B. "The Influence of Assortment Structure on Perceived Variety and Consumption Quantities," *The Journal of Consumer Research*. March 2004.

43 ABC Online Home. News in Science. "Chocolate Cake Addiction: It's Real." Reuters. April 24, 2004. Retrieved online May 26, 2004 from http://www.abc.net.au/science/news/stories/ s1091988.htm.

44 Hellmich, Nanci. "10 Ways to Make It a Habit to Eat Less, Eat Better and Exercise More," *USA Today*. January 6, 2004.

45 Parker-Pope, Tara. "The Diet that Works: What Science Tells Us About Weight Loss," *Wall Street Journal*. April 22, 2003.

46 Jakicic, J.M., Wing, R.R., Butler, B.A., & Robertson, R.J. "Prescribing Exercise in Multiple Short Bouts Versus One Continuous Bout: Effects on Adherence, Cardio Respiratory Fitness, and Weight Loss in Overweight Women." *International Journal of Obesity and Related Metabolic Disorders*, pp. 19, 893-901. 1995.

47 "How Much Exercise Is Enough?" Retrieved online June 24, 2004, from http://www.mayoclinic.com/invoke.cfm?objectid=02ACDB54-6F65-438B-9E7613BC252B0842.

48 Fitness Fundamentals. Developed by the President's Council on Physical Fitness and Sports. Retrieved online June 2, 2004, from http://www.hoptechno.com/book11.htm.

49 Hellmich, Nanci. "Walking Off 'Secret Flab,'" *USA Today*. January 15, 2003.

50 Medline Plus. "Muscle Atrophy." Retrieved online June 3, 2004, from http://www.nlm.nih.gov/medlineplus/ency/ article/003188.htm.

51 "Exercise Fuels the Brain's Stress Buffers," APA online, Psychology in Daily Life. Retrieved online June 3, 2004, from http://helping.apa.org/daily/neurala.html.

52 "Bulk Up Your Brain," REV, p. 19, Retrieved online from www.cnn.com/health. March and April 2004.

53 Wilmore, J. "Exercise, Obesity and Weight Control," Retrieved online June 3, 2004, from http://www.fitness.gov/activity/ activity7/obesity/obesity.html.

54 The American Council on Exercise. "Fit Facts: Can Exercise Reduce Your Risk of Catching a Cold?" Updated October 1, 2004. Retrieved online at http://www.acefitness.org/fitfacts/fitfacts_ display.cfm?itemid=79.

55 "Aerobic Exercise: Why and How?" From Mayoclinic.com. Special to CNN.com Health Library. April 1, 2003. Retrieved online June 24, 2004, from http://www.cnn.com/ HEALTH/library/EP/00002.html.

56 Quiz taken from www.loseitforlife.com.

57 Atlantic Health Science Corporation. "My Heart, I Take Care of It." Retrieved online June 3, 2004, from http://www.ahsc.health.nb.ca/hearthealth/highriskactivities.shtml.

58 Fitness Fundamentals. Developed by the President's Council on Physical Fitness and Sports. Retrieved online June 2, 2004, from http://www.hoptechno.com/book11.htm.

59 Information taken from www.loseitforlife.com.

60 Pierson, Vicki. "Starting an Exercise Program." Retrieved online June 3, 2004, from http://www.primusweb.com/ fitnesspartner/library/activity/startexercise.htm.

61 Stefano, Michael. "When It Comes to Exercise, Less Is More." Retrieved online June 3, 2004, from http://www.seekwellness.com/fitness/less_is_more.htm.

62 Bumgardner, Wendy. "What Is Planter Fasciitis and Heel Spur?" Retrieved online June 3, 2004, from http://walking.about.com/cs/heelpain/f/heelpain.htm.

63 "Walking, a Step in the Right Direction." NIH Publication No. 01-4155. March 2001. Retrieved online June 3, 2004, from http://www.niddk.nih.gov/health/nutrit/walking/walkingbro/walking.htm#okaywalk.

64 Gorrell, Carin. "Sarah Ferguson, The Duchess Weighs In," *Psychology Today*, p. 35. January-February 2002.

65 Mintle, Dr. Linda. Story adapted from *A Daughter's Journey Home*. Nashville, TN: Integrity Publishers, 2004.

66 Beck, A.T., Rush, A.J. , Shaw, B.F., & Emory, G. *Cognitive Therapy of Depression*. New York: Guilford. 1979.

67 Socrates. Quote. *Psychology Today*, p. 43. Retrieved online June 11, 2004, from http://www.famousquotes.com/ Search.php?search=Socrates&LastName=&FirstName=&field=LastName&paint=1&cat=&first=50.

68 Stuart, R. "Do Intimate Partners Help or Hinder Weight Loss?" *Psychology Today*. January/February 2002.

69 Ibid.

Appendices

Food Journal

Name: _____

Date: _____

When I ate	Where I ate	What I ate	How much I ate	Was I hungry?

Physical Versus Emotional Hunger Chart

When reviewing what you have eaten, it is important to be honest with yourself in order to find out whether it was physical hunger or an emotional feeling that triggered you to eat. Ask yourself the following three questions:

1. Was I experiencing physical or emotional hunger?
2. Before I ate, how did I feel?
3. After I ate, how did I feel?

Physical or emotional hunger?	Before I ate, I felt:	After I ate, I felt:

— APPENDIX C —

Glycemic Food Index[1]

BAKERY PRODUCTS	GI
Sponge cake	66
Pound cake	77
Danish	84
Muffin	88
Flan	93
Angel food cake	95
Croissant	96
Doughnut	108
Waffle	109

BREADS	GI
Oat bran bread	68
Mixed grain bread	69
Pumpernickel bread	71
White pita	82
Cheese pizza	86
Hamburger bun	87
Rye flour bread	92
Semolina bread	92
Oat kernel bread	93
Whole wheat bread	99
Melba toast	100
White bread	101
Plain bagel	103
Kaiser rolls	104
Bread stuffing	106
Gluten-free wheat bread	129
French baguette	136

BREAKFAST CEREALS	GI
Rice bran	27
Kellogg's All-Bran®	60
Oatmeal, non-instant	70
Special K®	77
Honey Smacks®	78
Oat bran	78
Kellogg's Meuslix®	80
Kellogg's Mini-Wheats® (unfrosted)	81
Multi-Bran Chex®	83
Kellogg's Just Right®	84
Life®	94
Grape-Nuts®	96
Post Shredded Wheat®	99
Cream of Wheat®	100
Golden Grahams®	102
Puffed wheat	105
Cheerios®	106
Corn bran	107
Total®	109
Rice Krispies®	117
Corn Chex®	118
Cornflakes	119
Crispix®	124
Rice Chex®	127

CEREAL GRAINS	GI
Pearled barley	36
Rye	48
Wheat kernels	59
Rice, instant	65
Bulgur	68
Rice, parboiled	68
Cracked barley	72
Wheat, quick cooking	77
Buckwheat	78
Brown rice	79
Wild rice	81
White rice	83
Couscous	93
Rolled barley	94
Mahatma Premium rice	94
Taco shells	97
Cornmeal	98
Millet	101
Tapioca, boiled with milk	115

COOKIES	GI
Oatmeal cookies	79
Shortbread	91
Arrowroot	95
Graham crackers	106
Vanilla Wafers®	110
Biscotti	113

CRACKERS	GI
Breton® wheat crackers	96
Stoned wheat thins	96
Rice cakes	110

[1] Glycemic Index numbers are provided by the World Health Organization.

DAIRY FOODS | GI

Low-fat yogurt, artificially sweetened	20
Chocolate milk, artificially sweetened	34
Whole milk	39
Soy milk	43
Fat-free milk	46
Low-fat yogurt, fruit flavored	47
Low-fat ice cream	71
Ice cream	87

FRUIT & FRUIT PRODUCTS | GI

Cherries	32
Grapefruit	36
Peach	40
Dried apricots	43
Fresh apricots	43
Canned peaches	43
Orange	47
Pear	47
Plum	55
Apple	56
Apple juice	57
Grapes	62
Canned pears	63
Raisins	64
Pineapple juice	66
Grapefruit juice	69
Fruit cocktail	79
Kiwifruit	83
Mango	86
Banana	89
Canned apricots, in syrup	91
Pineapple	94

Watermelon	103

LEGUMES | GI

Soybeans, boiled	23
Red lentils, boiled	36
Kidney beans, boiled	42
Green lentils, boiled	42
Butter beans, boiled	44
Yellow split peas, boiled	45
Baby lima beans, frozen	46
Chickpeas	47
Navy beans, boiled	54
Pinto beans	55
Black-eyed peas	59
Canned chickpeas	60
Canned pinto beans	64
Canned baked beans	69
Canned kidney beans	74
Canned green lentils	74
Fava beans	113

PASTA | GI

Protein-enriched spaghetti	38
Fettuccine	46
Vermicelli	50
Whole-grain spaghetti	53
Meat-filled ravioli	56
White spaghetti	59
Capellini	64
Macaroni	64
Linguine	65
Cheese tortellini	71
Durum spaghetti	78
Macaroni and cheese	92
Gnocchi	95
Brown rice pasta	113

ROOT VEGETABLES | GI

Sweet potato	63
Carrots, cooked	70
Yam	73
White potato, boiled	83
White potato, steamed	93
White potato, mashed	100
New potato	101
Rutabaga	103
Potato, boiled, mashed	104
French fries	107
Potatoes, instant	114
Potato, microwaved	117
Parsnips	139
Potato, baked	158

SNACK FOOD & CANDY | GI

Peanuts	21
Mars M&Ms® (peanut)	46
Mars Snickers® Bar	57
Mars Twix® Cookie Bars (caramel)	62
Chocolate bar, 1.5 oz	70
Jams and marmalades	70
Potato chips	77
Popcorn	79
Mars Kudos® Whole Grain Bars	87
Mars® Bar	91
Mars Skittles®	98
Life Savers®	100
Corn chips	105
Jelly beans	114
Pretzels	116
Dates	146

SOUPS	GI
Canned tomato soup	54
Canned lentil soup	63
Split pea soup	86
Black bean soup	92
Canned green pea soup	94

SUGARS	GI
Fructose	32
Lactose	65
Honey	83
High-fructose corn syrup	89
Sucrose	92
Glucose	137
Maltodextrin	150
Maltose	150

VEGETABLES	GI
Artichoke	<20
Argali	<20
Asparagus	<20
Broccoli	<20
Brussels sprouts	<20
Cabbage, all varieties	<20
Cauliflower	<20
Celery	<20
Cucumbers	<20
Escarole	<20
Eggplant	<20
Beet	<20
Chard	<20
Collard	<20
Kale	<20
Mustard	<20
Spinach	<20
Turnip	<20

Lettuce, all varieties	<20
Mushrooms, all varieties	<20
Okra	<20
Peanuts	<20
Peppers, all varieties	<20
Green beans	<20
Snow peas	<20
Spaghetti squash	<20
Young summer squash	<20
Watercress	<20
Wax beans	<20
Zucchini	<20
Tomatoes	23
Dried peas	32
Green peas	68
Sweet corn	78
Pumpkin	107

Two Weight-Loss Plans

For both plans, consult the following chart to plan meals; it's important to eat the number of servings listed for each food group. By eating the specified number, you will reduce carbohydrates but still get the proper amounts of food from other food groups to maintain a healthy weight-loss plan.

Food Group	1500-1800 Daily Calories			1800-2200 Daily Calories		
	Servings	Calories	Carbs(g)	Servings	Calories	Carbs(g)
Protein	9	495	0	14	890	0
Fats	6	270	0	8	360	0
Nuts	1	200	4	1	200	4
Vegetables	5	125	25	5	125	25
Starches	4	320	60	4	320	60
Fruits	2	120	30	2	120	30
Dairy	0.5	45	6	0.5	45	6
TOTAL		1575	125		2060	125

This plan is tailored to fit your calorie and carbohydrate needs while helping you lose about one to two pounds per week. Before you know it, you'll be losing the weight and loving your new low-carb lifestyle! Choose your desired number of daily calories and limit eating to the foods listed while observing the serving sizes listed in the appropriate column. All calorie levels are approximate. The following five-day meal plan allows 125 grams of carbs per day.

The Smart Low-Carb Weight-Loss Plan Menu
Recipes included on pages 252-259

MONDAY	Calorie Level 1500-1800	Calorie Level 1800-2200
Breakfast		
Fried Eggs in Vinegar*	1 serving	1 serving
Fat-free milk	½ cup	½ cup
Apple juice	½ cup	½ cup
Whole wheat bread	1 slice	1 slice
Butter spray, non-fat	1 tsp.	1 tsp.
Snack		
Nectarine, pear, or apple	1	1
Lunch		
Grilled chicken tenders	4 oz.	5 oz.
brushed w/ Italian dressing	1 tsp.	1 tbsp.
Red leaf lettuce	1 cup	1 cup
Carrot, shredded	¼ cup	¼ cup
Cucumber, sliced	½ cup	½ cup
Italian dressing	2 tsp.	2 tbsp.
Snack		
Walnuts	1 oz.	1 oz.
Dinner		
London broil	4 oz.	5 oz.
Spanish-style Green Beans*	1 serving	1 serving
Couscous	½ cup	½ cup
Snack		
Orange-Walnut Biscotti*	2	2
Total Calories	**1640**	**1880**
Total Carbs	**125**	**125**

TUESDAY	Calorie Level 1500-1800	Calorie Level 1800-2200
Breakfast		
Cherry Cream of Rye Cereal*	1 serving	1 serving
Fat-free milk	½ cup	½ cup
Turkey sausage	1 oz.	1 oz.
Snack		
Apple	1	1

Lunch

Tuna	3 oz.	4 oz.
Celery, chopped	¼ cup	¼ cup
Onion, chopped	¼ cup	¼ cup
Mayonnaise, reduced-fat	2 tbsp.	¼ cup
Green olives	10 small	10 small
Green leaf lettuce, torn	1 cup	1 cup
Whole wheat bread	1 slice	1 slice

Snack

Pecans	1 oz.	1 oz.

Dinner

Pork Chops Baked w/Cabbage and Cream*	1 serving	1 serving
Steamed butternut squash	½ cup	½ cup

Snack

Pumpernickel bread	1 slice	1 slice
Swiss cheese, reduced-fat	1 oz.	1 oz.
Butter spray, non-fat	1 tsp.	2 tsp.

Total Calories	**1670**	**1960**
Total Carbs	**127**	**127**

WEDNESDAY	Calorie Level 1500-1800	Calorie Level 1800-2200
Breakfast		
Scrambled egg	1	2
Orange juice	½ cup	½ cup
Rye toast	1 slice	1 slice
Butter spray, non-fat	1 tsp.	2 tsp.
Fat-free milk	½ cup	½ cup
Snack		
Kiwi	1	1
Lunch		
Salad of Lentils, cooked	½ cup	½ cup
Turkey breast, cooked and cubed	3 oz.	4 oz.
Carrots, sliced	½ cup	½ cup
Peppers, chopped	½ cup	½ cup
Peas, cooked	¼ cup	¼ cup
Olive oil	2 tsp.	1 tbsp.
Cheddar cheese, low-fat	½ oz.	½ oz.
Snack		
Brazil nuts	1 oz.	1 oz.

Dinner

Stir-Fried Chicken and Broccoli*	1 serving (4 oz. chicken)	1 serving (5 oz. chicken)

Snack

Pecan Muffins*	1	1
Butter	1 tsp.	2 tsp.
Total Calories	**1590**	**1890**
Total Carbs	**123**	**123**

THURSDAY	**Calorie Level 1500-1800**	**Calorie Level 1800-2200**

Breakfast

Pecan Muffins*	1	1
Cottage cheese, low-fat	2 tbsp.	6 tbsp.
Peach	1	1
Fat-free milk	½ cup	½ cup

Snack

Grapefruit	½	½

Lunch

Sandwich of two rice cakes topped w/ sardines or salmon, boneless, skinless	4 oz.	5 oz.
Cream cheese, low-fat	2 tbsp.	2 tbsp.
Tomato	2 slices	2 slices
Zucchini, sticks	½ cup	½ cup

Snack

Almonds	1 oz.	1 oz.

Dinner

Lamb chop topped	4 oz.	5 oz.
w/ garlic powder	⅛ tsp.	⅛ tsp.
Mint leaves	2 tsp.	1 tbsp.
Barley, cooked	½ cup	½ cup
Stewed tomatoes	1 cup	1 cup
Green beans, sautéed in olive oil	½ cup 2 tsp.	½ cup 3 tsp.

Snack

Whole wheat bread	1 slice	1 slice
Butter spray, non-fat	1 tsp.	2 tsp.
Chicken, sliced	1 oz.	2 oz.
Total Calories	**1700**	**1950**
Total Carbs	**122**	**122**

FRIDAY	Calorie Level 1500-1800	Calorie Level 1800-2200
Breakfast		
Sweet potato, cooked and topped	½ cup	½ cup
with walnut oil or canola oil	½ tsp.	1 tsp.
Walnuts, chopped	1 oz.	1 oz.
Coconut, shredded	1 tbsp.	2 tbsp.
Pineapple, crushed	¼ cup	¼ cup
Chicken breast, cooked	—	2 oz.
Fat-free milk	½ cup	½ cup
Lunch		
Salad of spinach	2 cups	2 cups
Chickpeas	½ cup	½ cup
Egg, hard-cooked	1	2
Artichoke hearts	½ cup	½ cup
Olive oil	2 tsp.	3 tsp.
Lemon juice	1 tbsp.	1 tbsp.
Whole wheat pita	½	½
Snack		
Monterey Jack cheese, low-fat	2 oz.	2 oz.
Dinner		
Breaded Baked Cod*	1 serving	1 serving
Red cabbage, sautéed in	½ cup	½ cup
sesame oil	1 tsp.	2 tsp.
Yellow squash, steamed	½ cup	½ cup
Butter spray, non-fat	1 tsp.	1 tsp.
Cantaloupe Sorbet*	1 serving	1 serving
Snack		
Popcorn, air-popped	3 cups	3 cups
Butter spray, non-fat	1 tsp.	2 tsp.
Monterey Jack cheese, reduced fat	2 oz.	2 oz.
Total Calories	**1640**	**1980**
Total Carbs	**124**	**124**

The Smart Low-Carb Weight-Loss Plan Recipes

Breaded Baked Cod with Tartar Sauce

Cantaloupe Sorbet

Cherry Cream of Rye Cereal

Fried Eggs with Vinegar

Orange Walnut Biscotti

Pecan Muffins

Pork Chops with Cabbage and Cream

Spanish-style Green Beans

Stir-fried Chicken with Broccoli

Breaded Baked Cod with Tartar Sauce

Serves: 4
Calories Per Serving: 268
Preparation Time: 30 minutes
Difficulty: Easy

Ingredients:
TARTAR SAUCE
½ cup reduced-fat mayonnaise or Lemonaise Lite®
1½ tbsp. lemon juice
1 tbsp. finely chopped dill or sweet pickles
2 tsp. mustard
2 tsp. capers, drained and chopped
2 tsp. chopped parsley (optional)

FISH
2 slices whole wheat bread
2 eggs or EggBeaters®
1 tbsp. water
1¼ lbs. cod or scrod fillet, cut into 1" pieces
½ tsp. salt (or salt substitute for a lower sodium choice)
¼ tsp. ground black pepper

Cooking Instructions:
1. To make the tartar sauce: In a small bowl, combine the mayonnaise, lemon juice, dill, mustard, capers, and parsley. Cover and refrigerate.
2. To make the fish: Preheat the oven to 400°F. Coat a baking sheet with cooking spray.
3. Place the bread in a food processor, and process into fine crumbs. Place in a shallow bowl. In another bowl, beat the eggs and water together. Season the fish with the salt and pepper.

4. Dip the fish into the egg mixture and then into the bread crumbs. Place fish on the prepared baking sheet. Generously coat the breaded fish with cooking spray.
5. Bake until fish pieces are opaque inside, about 10 minutes. Serve with the tartar sauce.

Per Serving Nutrition:

Fat:	10 g
Saturated fat:	2 g
Cholesterol:	174 mg
Carbs:	14 g
Protein:	30 g
Fiber:	1 g
Sodium:	734 mg*

*Using a salt substitute will lower the total sodium.

Tips:

· *If you buy your fish fresh, use within 2 days. Keep fish in its market wrapper in the refrigerator.*
· *Eating fish regularly offers many health benefits: Omega-3 fatty acids are believed to offer protection against heart disease, depression, and irregular menstrual cycles.*

Cantaloupe Sorbet

Ingredients:

4 frozen cantaloupes, slightly thawed
1 frozen banana, sliced
¼ cup Splenda®
1 tbsp. lime juice
2 tsp. grated lime peel
⅛-¼ tsp. ground cinnamon

Serves: 6
Calories Per Serving: 61
Preparation Time: 4-5 hours
Difficulty: Easy

Cooking Instructions:

1. In a food processor, combine the cantaloupe, banana, Splenda®, lime juice, lime peel, and cinnamon. Process until smooth.
2. Scrape into a shallow metal pan. Cover and freeze for 4 hours or overnight. Using a knife, break the mixture into chunks. Process briefly in a food processor to a smooth consistency before serving.

Per Serving Nutrition:

Fat:	0 g
Saturated Fat:	0 g
Cholesterol:	0 mg
Carbs:	15 g
Protein:	1 g
Fiber:	2 g
Sodium:	11 mg

Tips.

· *Cantaloupe is a powerful source of beta-carotene. Cantaloupe not only offers protection against cancer, it can help keep your skin lovely!*
· *To pick the juiciest, sweetest cantaloupe at the store, look for a melon that is heavy and without obvious injuries. The fragrance should be strong and sweet.*
· *Savory or lightly sweetened sorbets are customarily served either as a palate refresher between courses or as dessert.*

Cherry Cream of Rye Cereal

Serves: 4
Calories Per Serving: 208
Preparation Time: 10 minutes
Difficulty: Easy

Ingredients:

1¼ cup water
1¼ cup apple cider
¼ tsp. salt or salt substitute
1 cup cream of rye cereal
1 tbsp. low sugar or no sugar added cherry fruit spread
⅛ tsp. ground nutmeg
⅛ tsp. ground cardamom
1½ tbsp. chopped hazelnuts (optional)

Cooking Instructions:

1. Combine the water, cider, and salt in a saucepan and bring to a boil over medium heat. Stir in the cereal and reduce heat to low. Cook, uncovered, until thick, stirring occasionally, 3-5 minutes. Remove from heat and stir in the fruit spread.
2. Spoon into bowls and sprinkle with nutmeg, cardamom, and hazelnuts. Serve hot.

Per Serving Nutrition:

Fat:	1 g
Saturated Fat:	0 g
Cholesterol:	0 mg
Carbs:	45 g
Protein:	4 g
Fiber:	6 g
Sodium:	168 mg

Fried Eggs with Vinegar

Serves: 4
Calories Per Serving: 206
Preparation Time: 10 minutes
Difficulty: Easy

Ingredients:

2 tbsp. butter or non-fat butter spray
8 large eggs or EggBeaters®
1 tsp. salt or salt substitute
¼ tsp. ground black pepper
⅛ tsp. dried marjoram or basil
4 tsp. red wine vinegar
1 tsp. chopped parsley (optional)

Cooking Instructions:

1. Melt 1 tbsp. of butter in a large nonstick skillet over medium-low heat. Add the eggs, and sprinkle with the salt, pepper, and marjoram (work in batches if necessary). Cover and cook until the whites are set and yolks are almost set, 3 to 5 minutes. (For steam-basted eggs, add 1 tsp. of water to the pan and cover with a lid.)

2. Remove eggs to plates. Place the skillet over low heat and add the remaining 1 tbsp. of butter. Cook until the butter turns light brown, 1 to 2 minutes. Add the vinegar. Pour the vinegar mixture over the eggs. Sprinkle with parsley. Serve hot.

Per Serving Nutrition:

Fat:	16 g
Saturated Fat:	7 g
Cholesterol:	440 mg
Carbs:	1 g
Protein:	13 g
Fiber:	0 g
Sodium:	764 mg

Orange Walnut Biscotti

Serves: 24
Calories Per Serving: 76
Preparation Time: 1½ hours
Difficulty: Easy

Ingredients:

⅔ cup walnuts
¼ cup sugar
1¼ cup whole-grain pastry flour
¼ cup cornmeal
1 tsp. baking powder
¼ tsp. salt or salt substitute
¼ cup butter, softened or non-fat butter spray
¼ cup Splenda®
2 large eggs or EggBeaters®
2 tsp. grated orange peel
½ tsp. orange extract

Cooking Instructions:

1. In a food processor, combine the walnuts and 2 tablespoons of the sugar. Process just until walnuts are coarsely ground. Transfer to a large bowl and add the flour, cornmeal, baking powder, and salt. Stir until combined.
2. In a large bowl, and using an electric mixer, beat the butter, Splenda, and remaining 2 tablespoons of sugar until light and fluffy. Beat in the eggs, orange peel, and orange extract. Gradually beat in the flour mixture until dough is smooth and thick. Divide the dough into two equal-sized discs. Refrigerate for 30 minutes or until dough is firm.
3. Preheat the oven to 350°F. Coat a baking sheet with cooking spray.
4. Shape each disc into a 12" log. Place both logs on the prepared baking sheet. Bake for 25 to 30 minutes, or until golden brown. Remove the logs to wire racks to cool.
5. Cut each log on a slight diagonal into ½"-thick slices. Place the slices, cut side down, on the baking sheet and bake for 5 minutes. Turn the slices over, and bake for 5 minutes longer, or until dry. Remove biscotti to wire racks to cool.

Per Serving Nutrition:

Fat:	5 g
Saturated fat:	2 g
Cholesterol:	23 mg
Carbs:	8 g
Protein:	2 g
Fiber:	1 g
Sodium:	68 mg

Tips:

· *Walnuts are a good source of alpha-linolenic acid, which can reduce your risk of heart attack and stroke.*

Pecan Muffins

Ingredients:

1½ cups whole grain pastry flour
¼ cup soy flour
2½ tsp. baking powder
½ tsp. salt or salt substitute
½ tsp. ground nutmeg
½ cup toasted pecans, chopped
½ cup vegetable oil
½ cup low sugar or no sugar added apricot or peach fruit spread
 2 large eggs or EggBeaters®, lightly beaten
1½ tsp. vanilla extract
⅛ tsp. liquid stevia* or Splenda®
Available in most health-food stores

> Serves: 12
> Calories Per Serving:
>   One muffin, 218
> Preparation Time: 25 Minutes
> Difficulty: Easy

Cooking Instructions:

1. Place a rack in the middle position in the oven. Preheat the oven to 375°F. Coat a 12-cup muffin pan with cooking spray or line with paper cups.
2. In a large bowl, whisk together the pastry flour, soy flour, baking powder, salt, nutmeg, and pecans.
3. In a small bowl, combine the oil, fruit spread, eggs, vanilla extract, and stevia. Add to the flour mixture, stirring just until the dry ingredients are moistened.
4. Spoon into the prepared muffin cups until three-quarters full. Bake 12-14 minutes or until a toothpick inserted in the center of a muffin comes out clean. Serve warm.

Per Serving Nutrition:

Fat:	12 g
Saturated Fat:	1 g
Cholesterol:	35 mg
Carbs:	20 g
Protein:	4 g
Fiber:	3 g
Sodium:	193 mg

Tips:

· *Whole-wheat pastry flour is available at most health-food stores.*
· *Whole grains reduce your risk of heart disease, cancer, and other chronic illnesses. Always choose whole-grain breads and pasta over any made from refined white flour.*

Pork Chops Baked with Cabbage & Cream

Serves: 4
Calories Per Serving: 463
Preparation Time: 50 minutes
Difficulty: Average

Ingredients:

1 small head (1½ lbs.) green cabbage, cored and
    finely shredded
4 boneless pork chops (6 oz. each), each ¾" thick
½ tsp. salt or salt substitute
¼ tsp. ground black pepper
2 tsp. olive oil
½ cup half-and-half
1 tsp. caraway seeds
½ tsp. sweet Hungarian paprika
1 tsp. dried marjoram or thyme
½ cup (2 oz.) shredded low-fat Swiss cheese

Cooking Instructions:

1. Preheat the oven to 350°F.
2. Bring a large pot of salted water to a boil over high heat. Add the cabbage and cook
   until soft, 4-5 minutes. Drain in a colander and allow to dry on paper towels.
3. Season the meat with ¼ tsp. of the salt and pepper. Heat the oil in a large oven-
   proof skillet over high heat. Add the meat and cook just until browned, 1-2 minutes.
   Remove to a plate.
4. Discard any fat in the skillet and heat the skillet over low heat. Stir in the cabbage,
   half-and-half, caraway seeds, paprika, marjoram, and the remaining ¼ teaspoon
   of salt. Cook and stir until heated through, about 5 minutes. Remove from heat
   and place chops on a plate. Place cabbage in skillet and arrange the pork over the
   cabbage, adding any juices accumulated on the plate. Sprinkle with the cheese. Bake
   until a meat thermometer registers 160°F for medium-well, about 25 minutes.

Per Serving Nutrition:

Fat:	20 g
Saturated Fat:	9 g
Cholesterol:	165 mg
Carbs:	12 g
Protein:	53 g
Fiber:	4 g
Sodium:	460 mg

Tips:

· *Vegetables like cabbage help reduce your risk of
  heart disease, cancer, and stroke.*
· *Cabbage is also high in calcium, which protects
  bone density.*

Spanish-style Green Beans

Serves: 4
Calories Per Serving: 162
Preparation Time: 30 minutes
Difficulty: Easy

Ingredients:

16 oz. green beans, trimmed and
    cut into 2" lengths

3 tbsp. olive oil
1 onion, chopped
1 small green bell pepper, chopped
1 tomato (4 oz.), peeled, seeded, and coarsely chopped
2 cloves garlic, minced
¼ tsp. salt or salt substitute
⅛ tsp. ground black pepper
2-3 tbsp. coarsely chopped, pitted kalamata olives
2 tsp. drained capers (optional)

Cooking Instructions:

1. Combine the beans, oil, onion, bell pepper, tomato, garlic, salt, and black pepper in a saucepan over medium heat. Cook, stirring, until the vegetables start to sizzle, 2-3 minutes.
2. Reduce the heat to low, cover, and cook, stirring occasionally, until the beans are very tender but not falling apart, 20-25 minutes. Stir in olives and capers and heat for 1 minute. Serve warm, at room temperature, or chilled.

Per Serving Nutrition:

Fat:	12 g
Saturated Fat:	2 g
Cholesterol:	0 mg
Carbs:	13 g
Protein:	2 g
Fiber:	6 g
Sodium:	230 mg

Tips:

· *Eating more vegetables helps you feel full and satisfied longer.*
· *Fiber-rich foods, such as green beans, help to lower cholesterol levels.*

Stir-fried Chicken and Broccoli

Serves: 4
Calories Per Serving: 321
Preparation Time: 20 minutes
Difficulty: Easy

Ingredients:

½ cup chicken broth
3 tbsp. Chinese oyster sauce
2 tbsp. orange juice
1 tbsp. + 1½ tsp. low sodium soy sauce
2 cloves garlic, minced
2 tsp. fresh ginger, minced
1 tsp. sesame oil
¼ tsp. hot-pepper sauce (optional)
1 tbsp. cornstarch
1 tbsp. + 1½ tsp. cold water
3 tbsp. vegetable oil
1 lb. boneless, skinless chicken breasts, cut into thin strips

1 large bunch (2 lbs.) broccoli, cut into small florets
5 scallions, sliced
sesame seeds (optional)

Cooking Instructions:

1. In a small bowl, combine the broth, oyster sauce, orange juice, soy sauce, garlic, ginger, sesame oil, and hot-pepper sauce.
2. In a cup, dissolve the cornstarch in the cold water.
3. Heat the oil in a large wok or skillet over high heat until the oil just starts to smoke. Add the chicken and cook, stirring constantly, until it is no longer pink on the surface, about 30 seconds. Add the broccoli and cook, stirring constantly, until it turns bright green and the chicken is half-cooked, about 2 minutes.
4. Pour in the broth mixture and cook for 2 minutes, stirring frequently.
5. Stir in the scallions and cornstarch mixture. Cook and stir until the sauce comes to a boil and thickens, and the chicken is cooked through, about 1 minute.
6. Sprinkle with the sesame seeds.

Per Serving Nutrition:

Fat:	14 g
Saturated Fat:	1 g
Cholesterol:	66 mg
Carbs:	18 g
Protein:	34 g
Fiber:	8 g
Sodium:	692 mg

Tips:

· *Avoid buying broccoli with yellow tips. If it isn't fresh, it won't taste as good.*
· *Eating broccoli and other cruciferous vegetables regularly will help lower your risk of cancer.*

The Walker's Weight-Loss Plan

To lose weight, your goal is to burn more calories a day than you eat. Remember these six essential factors:

1. CONTROL YOUR CALORIES. If you exercise three days a week or less and do only minimal daily activity, a good daily calorie level is 1,350. You could lose up to two pounds per week at this level. If you exercise four days a week by walking, jogging, or doing in-home cardio exercise, you could increase your calorie level to 1,600 each day and still lose up to two pounds per week.

2. INCREASE YOUR FIBER INTAKE. Choose high-fiber foods over low-fiber foods. Each gram of fiber eaten can cancel out nine calories from your daily caloric intake! Try high-fiber multigrain breakfast cereals, barley, whole-wheat bread, and fruits such as pears and raspberries. Eat four servings a week of legumes such as beans, peas, and lentils. Some ideas for how to get lentils into your diet include bean or lentil salad, vegetable chili, low-fat refried beans, baked beans, and bean burritos.

3. REPLACE HIGH-FAT FOODS WITH CHOICES THAT ARE LOWER IN FAT. Read all food labels and try to stay within the range of no more than 25 percent of your calories coming from fat. Good choices include: avocados, olives, peanut butter, and nuts. Try olive and canola oil for cooking, in your salad dressings, or on your bread. Favor unsalted nuts over chips or other snack foods.

4. EAT AT LEAST ONE FIBER-RICH FRUIT OR VEGETABLE EACH DAY. The choices are many! Carrots, sweet potatoes, squash, tomatoes, cantaloupes, apricots, oranges, grapefruit, papayas, red peppers, or broccoli.

5. ELIMINATE OR REDUCE SUGAR. Remember that too much sugar turns to fat!

6. REDUCE SALT. According to the USDA, too much sodium can elevate blood pressure and lead to stroke. Too much salt can also cause water retention. Avoid canned or pre-packaged foods in favor of the frozen or fresh variety. Read all food labels to make sure the sodium content is within reasonable limits. If you're trying to lose weight, you should have no more than 2,000 mg of sodium per day. Salt is literally in everything, so be careful when eating out and ask your waiter or waitress to "hold the salt" on your order.

The Walker's Weight-Loss Plan Menu

*Recipes included on pages 265-268

MONDAY

Breakfast
½ grapefruit
1 slice whole wheat toast
1 tbsp. low sugar or no-sugar-
 added fruit spread

Mid-morning Snack
¾ cup Concord grape juice
1 cup oatmeal
1 cup fat-free milk

Lunch
1 cup black bean soup
1 wedge cornbread
1 cup spinach salad topped with
 ½ cup orange sections

Mid-afternoon Snack
1 oz. reduced-fat cheddar cheese
2 tbsp. walnuts
1 apple

Dinner
1 cup cooked whole wheat pasta
 shells tossed with 1 tbsp. olive
 oil and 2 cloves garlic
1 cup broccoli
½ cup red bell pepper slices

Evening Snack
1 cup reduced-sodium tomato juice
4 whole wheat crackers

Nutrition Information:
Calories:	1506
Fat:	45 g
Saturated Fat:	10 g
Fiber:	23 g
Sodium:	2168 mg

Tips:
· *To find whole-wheat bread, check the ingredients list; the first ingredient should be "whole-wheat flour."*
· *Concord grape juice has almost five times the antioxidant power of orange juice.*
· *Today's improved reduced-fat cheeses taste as good as the real thing.*
· *Eating mini-meals (at breakfast, midmorning snack, lunch, mid-afternoon snack, dinner, and evening snack) may help prevent weight gain.*
· *Chop garlic, then let it "rest" for 15 minutes before cooking so that healing phytochemicals have a chance to develop.*
· *Processed tomato products are concentrated sources of lycopene, a likely prostate cancer fighter.*

TUESDAY

Breakfast
½ whole wheat English muffin
1 tsp. trans-free margarine or
 non-fat butter spray
1 poached or hard-cooked egg or
 EggBeaters®
1 pear

Nutrition Information:
Calories:	1506
Fat:	38 g
Saturated fat:	10 g
Fiber:	21 g
Sodium:	1337 mg

Mid-morning Snack
½ cup low-fat vanilla yogurt
½ cup low-fat granola

Lunch
2 slices whole wheat bread with
2 oz. reduced-fat mozzarella
cheese and 1 roasted bell pepper
(packed in water) or fresh
Basil leaves

Mid-afternoon Snack
¼ cup hummus
½ cup cucumber slices

Dinner
3 oz. poached salmon
1 cup brown rice
½ cup no-salt-added stewed
tomatoes
1 cup steamed kale

Evening Snack
½ cup calcium-fortified orange
juice
1 banana

WEDNESDAY

Breakfast
¾ cup hot whole wheat cereal
½ cup frozen blueberries, thawed
1 cup fat-free milk

Mid-morning Snack
1 slice toasted whole wheat raisin
bread
1 tbsp. natural or low-fat peanut
butter

Lunch
1 small bean burrito
8 grape tomatoes, halved and
tossed with 2 oz. crumbled
reduced-fat feta cheese

Mid-afternoon Snack
1 serving Papaya Power Shake*

Tips:
· Check ingredients lists; look for margarine
without the words "partially hydrogenated."
· Mix your yogurt and granola the night before
and freeze. By the time you get ready to eat
your snack at work, it should be defrosted.
· Choosing fruits and vegetables with vivid colors
helps you zero in on the nutrient powerhouses.
· The Italian section of the ethnic food aisle has
ready-to-eat jarred red bell peppers. If you're
concerned with sodium levels, and the sodium is
high on the pre-prepared items, stick with fresh
vegetables.
· Look for calcium-fortified red grapefruit juice
too.
· Poaching is very healthy and quite easy. Bring
water (enough to cover the fish), a bay leaf, a
lemon slice, and a little salt or salt substitute to
a boil in a skillet. Lower to a simmer, then
place the fish in the liquid. Cook gently for
about 8 minutes or until cooked through.

Nutrition Information:
Calories:	1529
Fat:	45 g
Saturated Fat:	15 g
Fiber:	30 g
Sodium:	2609 mg

Tips:
· Blueberries are the top source of antioxidants
among all fruits and vegetables.
· Choose natural peanut butter to avoid trans-
fatty acids.
· Healthy microwavable burritos are available in
the frozen food case.

Dinner
2 oz. roast chicken breast
1 cup mashed butternut squash
1 cup brussels sprouts
½ cup corn kernels mixed with
  ¼ cup cooked barley and
  2 tsp. canola oil

Evening Snack
1 extra large baked apple with
  2 tsp. honey or brown sugar

THURSDAY

Breakfast
½ toasted whole wheat bagel
  topped with ¼ cup reduced-fat
  ricotta cheese
3 finely chopped prunes

Mid-morning Snack
1 cup low-fat plain yogurt with
  ½ sliced banana and 1 tbsp.
  chopped walnuts

Lunch
Pasta salad made with:
1 cup cooked whole wheat rotini
  or pasta spirals
½ cup broccoli
½ cup yellow bell pepper
½ tomato, chopped
1 tbsp. olive oil
1 tsp. vinegar

Mid-afternoon Snack
2 rye crispbread sheets
2 tbsp. light cream cheese
½ cup frozen strawberries, thawed

Dinner
1 serving Carrot Soup with Lime
  and Chiles*
6 large shrimp broiled with 1 tbsp.
  of low-sodium teriyaki sauce
1 cup cooked whole wheat couscous
½ cup green peas

Nutrition Information:
Calories:	1586
Fat:	46 g
Saturated fat:	15 g
Fiber:	28 g
Sodium:	1803 mg

Tips:
· *For an extra flavor boost, try lemon or orange flavored prunes.*
· *Lightly toasting walnuts in a small skillet for a few minutes really brings out the flavor.*
· *If you are cooking for just one or two, it makes sense to grab vegetables from the supermarket salad bar.*
· *Look for brands with 4-5 grams of fiber per two-cracker serving, such as WASA Fiber Rye Crispbread and Natural Rye crisp crackers.*

Evening Snack
> ½ cup pear slices tossed with
> ½ oz. blue cheese or brie

FRIDAY

Breakfast
> 1 cup fat-free milk
> 1 Raisin Bran Muffin*
> ½ cup grapes

Mid-morning Snack
> 1 slice toasted cracked-wheat bread
> topped with ½ mashed banana
> 1 tangerine

Lunch
> 1 cup tabbouleh
> 1 raw carrot
> 1 whole wheat pita round

Mid-afternoon Snack
> 1 cup reduced-sodium tomato
> soup made with ⅓ cup fat-free
> milk
> 8 rye crisp rounds

Dinner
> 1 serving Spicy Lentils*
> ½ cup brown rice
> 1 cup steamed spinach mixed with
> ½ cup diced canned tomatoes

Evening Snack
> 1 brown rice cake
> ½ oz. reduced-fat cheddar cheese

Nutritional Information:

Calories:	1523
Fat:	22 g
Saturated fat:	3.8 g
Fiber:	26 g
Sodium:	2869 mg

Tips:
- *Make a batch of tabbouleh from a mix (available in the rice aisle), but substitute lemon juice for some oil.*
- *Rice cakes have exploded with flavors in the past few years, so take your pick.*
- *In the winter, canned tomatoes have far more flavor than fresh.*
- *The instant versions of bean soup that require only boiling water are great! But watch the sodium levels!*

The Walker's Weight-Loss Plan Menu Recipes

Carrot Soup with Lime and Chiles

Papaya Power Shake

Raisin Bran Muffins

Spicy Lentils

Carrot Soup with Lime and Chiles

Serves: 4
Calories Per Serving: 130
Preparation Time: 35 minutes
Difficulty: Easy

Ingredients:

1 tbsp. olive or canola oil
1 large onion, finely chopped
2 large cloves garlic, chopped*
½ lb. peeled, ready-to-eat baby carrots
½ cup uncooked instant brown rice
2 cans (14½ oz. each) fat-free, reduced-sodium chicken broth
1 cup water
½ tsp. salt or salt substitute
1 tbsp. chopped green chilies
juice of 1 lime (about 2 tbsp.)
1 tbsp. prepared chopped garlic can be substituted

Cooking Instructions:

1. Heat the oil in a large nonstick saucepan over medium heat. Add the onion and sauté for 3 minutes. Add the garlic and sauté 1 minute longer.
2. Add the carrots, rice, broth, water, and salt to the saucepan. Bring to a boil, then reduce the heat to medium low. Simmer, partially covered, for 20 minutes, or until the carrots are tender. Stir in the chilies and lime juice.
3. Puree the soup in a food processor or blender. The best method is to place half of the solids in the food processor and add just enough of the broth to liquefy the carrots and rice. Add the rest of the solids, then stir the puree back into the remaining broth.
4. Reheat if necessary. Serve warm. If desired, garnish with chopped fresh cilantro, thinly sliced scallions, a dollop of plain yogurt, and additional chopped chili peppers.

Per Serving Nutrition:

Fat:	4 g
Saturated Fat:	0.5 g
Cholesterol:	0 mg
Carbs:	21 g
Protein:	5 g

Fiber: 3 g
Sodium: 717 mg*

*Using a salt substitute will lower the total sodium.

Papaya Power Shake

Ingredients:

1 papaya, peeled, seeded, and cut up
1 cup low-fat plain yogurt
½ banana
½ cup no sugar added pineapple chunks
½ tsp. dried mint
4 ice cubes, slightly crushed

Serves: 4
Calories Per Serving: 88
Preparation Time: 5 minutes
Difficulty: Easy

Cooking Instructions:

Combine all ingredients in a blender and process until smooth.

Per Serving Nutrition:

Fat:	1 g
Saturated Fat	1 g
Cholesterol:	4 mg
Carbs:	17 g
Protein:	4 g
Fiber:	2 g
Sodium:	44 mg

Tip:

· *This shake also works well with canned mango spears, which are available in the produce aisle of most supermarkets.*

Raisin Bran Muffins

Ingredients:

1 cup low-fat buttermilk
¾ cup bud-style bran cereal
   (such as Bran Buds™, 100% Bran™, or Fiber One™)
½ cup golden raisins
½ cup shredded carrots
1 egg or EggBeaters®
⅓ cup honey
¼ cup canola oil
1 tsp. vanilla extract
1 cup whole wheat flour
1 tsp. baking soda
1 tsp. ground cinnamon
1 tbsp. honey-crunch wheat germ (optional)

Serves: 12 muffins
Calories per Serving: 164
Preparation Time: 45 minutes
Difficulty: Easy

Cooking Instructions:

1. Preheat the oven to 425°F. Line a 12-cup muffin pan with paper liners; coat the papers with cooking spray.
2. In a medium bowl, combine the buttermilk, cereal, raisins, carrots, egg, honey, oil, and vanilla extract. Let it stand for 15 minutes.
3. In a large bowl, combine the flour, baking soda, and cinnamon. Make a well in the center and add the buttermilk mixture all at once. Stir just enough to moisten the flour.
4. Divide the batter evenly among the muffin cups. Sprinkle the tops with wheat germ. Bake for 15-20 minutes, or until a toothpick inserted in the center comes out clean.

Per Serving Nutrition:

Fat:	6 g
Saturated Fat:	1 g
Cholesterol:	18 mg
Carbs:	28 g
Protein:	4 g
Fiber:	3 g
Sodium:	131 mg

Tips:

· *If you can't find high-fiber/low-sugar oat bran muffins, these are a great substitute.*
· *Make a double batch of these for fast breakfast treats.*

Spicy Lentils

Ingredients:

1 tbsp. canola oil
1 cup onion, finely chopped
2 tsp. ground ginger
1 tsp. ground cumin
1 cup dried red or brown lentils
3 cups water
¾ tsp. salt or salt substitute
2 tbsp. fresh cilantro, finely chopped
1 tbsp. lemon juice

Serves: 4
Calories Per Serving: 167
Preparation Time: 35 minutes
Difficulty: Easy

Cooking Instructions:

1. Heat the oil in a medium saucepan. Add the onion and sauté, stirring often, for 5 minutes or until tender. Stir in the ginger and cumin and sauté 30 seconds longer.
2. Add the lentils, water, and salt. Heat to a boil. Reduce the heat to low and simmer, partially covered, for 15 minutes.
3. If the lentils are tender, uncover and gently boil until most of the liquid evaporates. If the lentils are too hard, continue to cook, partially covered, ten minutes longer or until lentils are tender.*
4. Remove lentils from heat and stir in cilantro and lemon juice. Serve warm. Serve this soupy, stew-like dish in a shallow bowl over brown rice.

Cooking time for lentils can vary from 15 minutes to as long as 1 hour, depending on the type and age of the lentils. Red lentils (which turn yellow when cooked) cook very quickly because they are split, and after 15 to 20 minutes, they soften to a puree. Brown lentils hold their shape better but can take longer to cook.

Per Serving Nutrition:

Fat:	4 g
Saturated Fat:	0 g
Cholesterol:	0 mg
Carbs:	25 g
Protein:	10 g
Fiber:	6 g
Sodium:	406 mg

— Appendix E —

Physical Exercises

The Ten-Minute Workout

Tone up and trim down! Set aside a few minutes several times a day for these great exercises and you'll shed those excess pounds! Remember: keep your routine short and simple. Have weights handy and do any combination of these simple exercises at structured or random times. Over time you will notice better muscle tone and increased strength.

Lean muscle has very little fat and burns more calories than underdeveloped muscle. Keeping your muscles lean requires physical resistance that can be achieved by lifting light weights several minutes daily. If you have your doctor's permission, you can follow this simple workout.

1. BICEPS. You need three-pound, four-pound, or five-pound hand weights, or equivalent weights using water or sand-filled plastic bottles. A half-gallon container filled with water weighs about four and a half pounds. A sand-filled plastic half-gallon container weighs seven and a half pounds. Double these weight amounts for a gallon size. You do not have to fill the containers completely; approximate and determine a comfortable weight.

Keeping your arms down at your sides, hold one weight in each hand against each thigh. Slowly lift your arms parallel to the floor or ground. Slowly return your arms to the original position. Repeat gradually five to ten times.

Hold weights next to your thighs (starting position). Bend your arms up and then continue the motion to lift weights over your head. Repeat slowly five to ten times.

2. TRICEPS. Hold weights next to your thighs. Slowly raise both forearms so they are parallel to the floor or ground and make a 90-degree angle. Slowly lower weights to the starting position. Return to the 90-degree angle and repeat movement five to ten times.

Hold weights with your arms extended downward. Slowly shrug your shoulders (lifting weights with shoulder muscles). Repeat five to ten times.

3. LEGS. Hold weights against thighs. Slowly squat, then rise. (Do not squat to a position that is uncomfortable.) Repeat five to ten times.

Using weights, bend your arms up and hold weights against your chest. Slowly slide one leg forward as far as you comfortably can while keeping the other leg stationary; then return your leg to the starting position. Repeat movement with other leg. Repeat five to ten times per leg.

4. ARM CURL. Hold weights and extend arms downward at sides with palms facing forward. Alternately curl weights in each arm upward while keeping elbows at the same level each time. Slowly repeat five to ten times per each arm.

5. ANKLE WEIGHTS. Strap a light ankle weight on each leg, and do leg lifts standing or sitting; move legs to the side one at a time while standing, or together when sitting. Slowly repeat movements five to ten times. Do not overdo this exercise!

The In-Home Cardio Routine

If you prefer to exercise at home or need to stay indoors because of bad weather, try this in-home cardio routine. Set aside twenty to thirty minutes. It's okay if you're not able to go the full thirty-minute session at first. Remember, any movement is better than none!

Begin at a level you can maintain. Then, slowly add a few minutes to each session. Do each of the moves for two to three minutes, alternating options throughout. Rotate your schedule between doing this routine two days a week and walking the other two days. This rotation schedule will provide variety as well as alternate the workout for your muscles.

Eight options

1. MARCHING OR RUNNING IN PLACE. This is great as a warm-up before your routine starts. Be sure to work your whole body by pumping your arms and getting your knees nice and high.

2. CROSSOVERS. Stand and place your hands behind your head. Lift your left knee up to your right elbow and then lower it again. Do the same with the other side of your body. Repeat for two to three minutes. (You'll find this also works on your waistline!)

3. KICKS. Stand and bring your fists to the level of your chest (as if you are blocking an imaginary opponent). Raise your left knee to your waist and then kick your lower leg forward to extend your leg. Tighten your abs as you kick in the air. Lower and repeat with the other leg. Repeat for two to three minutes, continuing to switch legs. (This move is called a front kick in kickboxing.)

4. PUNCHES. Bend your knees slightly and punch forward with your

right arm (imagine you're boxing). Release and repeat with your left arm. Do this exercise for two to three minutes. (You'll find this routine great for toning your arms.)

5. JUMP ROPE. Skipping rope is great for the whole body. To bring in variety, try jogging or skipping like a boxer as you jump. Continue for two to three minutes.

6. JUMP SQUATS. Stand with your feet together and arms at your sides. Then squat like you are going to sit in a chair. Keep your abs pulled in and your torso straight. Jump up into the air, land, and repeat. Slightly bend your knees as you land to minimize the impact. Continue for two to three minutes. (You may find this exercise challenging, but do the best you can. You'll find it's great for your rear end!)

7. WAIST TWISTS. Imagine you're skiing down a hill. Place your feet together and lightly jump and pivot your knees and toes to the right. Lift your right elbow out to the right (at shoulder height) and extend your left arm out to the left at the same time. Repeat the move in the opposite direction without lowering your arms. Continue for two to three minutes.

8. JACK-IN-THE-BOX. Squat like you're sitting in a chair, keeping your feet together. Then jump up and spread your hands and feet out so you make an X with your arms and legs (like a jumping jack). Repeat for two to three minutes. (You'll find this exercise great for your inner and outer thighs!)

Practice Relaxation

Relaxation is a great substitute for overeating. The problem is many of us don't know how to relax. We become fidgety and bored and end up reaching for food. When a highly stressful period hits (at work, for instance), put a time limit on the amount of time you will give to thinking about it. To relax in spite of the stress, build into your day moments of distraction and practice relaxation exercises.

Deep Muscle Relaxation

There are a number of easy relaxation exercises you can do to de-stress without using food. If you carry stress in your physical body, deep muscle relaxation may be for you. It's easy to do. Just clench your fist, hold it tense, and then relax it. Do this again and then move on to another muscle in your body. In deep muscle relaxation, you are taking each muscle group, tensing it, and then releasing it. This exercise teaches you the difference between tension and relaxation. Practice deep muscle relaxation up to thirty minutes a day if you carry a lot of tension in your body. You can practice in the morning when you wake up and start your day refreshed, or you can practice in the evening before bedtime to calm yourself down. The more you practice, the easier it will become for you to relax.

Deep Breathing

Another easy technique is deep breathing. Slowly inhale and breathe deeply from your abdomen—now you are deep breathing. When we get tense, we tend to take short, shallow breaths from our chest. But deep breathing is slow and originates in the abdomen. When you feel stressed and want to eat, take a few deep breaths and relax your body. Do this several times a day if need be. The great thing about deep breathing is you can do it anywhere—in traffic, at work, in the house, or even in the park.

Lose Weight in Just Thirty Days[2]

Walking is easy, cheap, convenient, and not likely to result in injury. Rebecca Gorrell, director of fitness and movement therapy at Canyon Ranch in Tucson, Arizona, helped develop three walking workouts guaranteed to have you dropping pounds in just thirty days.

The higher the intensity of your walk, the more calories you'll burn. But how do you know at what intensity you're working? An easy, low-tech method to use is the Borg Scale for Rate of Perceived Exertion (RPE). No arithmetic or heart-rate monitors are needed.

To use it, monitor your body and consider how hard you are working. Is your breathing heavy? Are you sweating? Do your muscles feel warm? Are they burning? Now, rate how you feel.

Borg Scale for Rate of Perceived Exertion (RPE)

6	Very, very light
7	(lounging on
8	the couch)
9	Very light
10	(puttering around the house)
11	Fairly light
12	(strolling leisurely)
13	Somewhat hard
14	(normal walking)
15	Hard
16	(walking as if in a hurry)
17	Very hard
18	(jogging/running)
19	Very, very hard
20	(sprinting)

Borg RPE scale, © Gunnar Borg, 1970, 1985, 1994, 1998.

---

[2] All walking plans are adapted from www.loseitforlife.com

Week #	Time	Length	Plateau-Busting Plan	RPE*
Week 1	35 min.	5 days	Warm-up (5 min.)	10-11
			Normal walk (5 min.)	13
			Speed up (5 min.)	15
			Recovery (10 min.)	13
			Speed up (5 min.)	15
			Cooldown (5 min.)	0-11
Week 2	35 min.	5 days	Warm-up (5 min.)	10-11
			Normal walk (5 min.)	13
			Speed up (5 min.)	16
			Recovery (10 min.)	13
			Speed up (5 min.)	16
			Cooldown (5 min.)	10-11
Week 3	45 min.	5 days	Warm-up (5 min.)	10-11
			Normal walk (5 min.)	13
			Speed up (5 min.)	16
			Recovery (8 min.)	13
			Speed up (5 min.)	16
			Recovery (7 min.)	13
			Speed up (5 min.)	16
			Cooldown (5 min.)	10-11
Week 4	45 min.	5 days	Warm-up (5 min.)	10-11
			Speed up (5 min.)	16
			Recovery (5 min.)	13
			Speed up (5 min.)	16
			Recovery (5 min.)	13
			Speed up (5 min.)	16
			Recovery (5 min.)	13
			Speed up (5 min.)	16
			Cooldown (5 min.)	10-11

*RPE is Rate of Perceived Exertion

Plan #1: The Plateau-Busting Plan

Have you stopped losing weight even though you regularly walk? Perhaps you've reached a plateau. Try adding intervals to your program or increase your pace. Set new goals to achieve increased weight loss.

Plan #2: The Muscle-Toning Circuit Plan

Shape your muscles when you walk! This plan is for you if you want firmer muscles, need some variety, and have been walking regularly. Try the different techniques in the muscle-toning circuit to firm up your muscles (toning exercises follow chart).

Week #	Time	Length	(See below for exercise descriptions.) Muscle-Toning Circuit Plan	RPE*
Week 1	30 min.	5 days	2 min. each segment	13-15
Week 2	40 min.	5 days	3 min. each segment	13-15
Week 3	50 min.	5 days	4 min. each segment	13-15
Week 4	60 min.	5 days	5 min. each segment	13-15

*RPE is Rate of Perceived Exertion

Exercise Descriptions

1. HILLS OR STAIR CLIMBING firms up the fronts and backs of your calves and thighs.
2. RACE WALKING shapes your abdomen and upper back muscles. You race walk by taking shorter, quicker steps. Use your arms for more power, keeping them bent at 85- to 90-degree angles.
3. THE BUTT SQUEEZE tones the gluteus muscles. Use your normal walking form, but as you press off the toes of your back leg, squeeze your buttocks firmly. Be careful not to tense your lower back.
4. BACKWARD WALKING strengthens the back and abdomen. Do your walk backwards. Tuck your belly in and put your hands on

your hips. You'll find your abs and back doing all the work. For safety, try this only on a level track or path.

Plan #3: The Incline Walking Plan

Take your walking exercise to the next level and burn up to 50 percent more calories in the process by raising the incline on the treadmill in your home or gym. Follow this routine every other day, and you will want to rest your muscles between these workouts.

STEP ONE: Before adding your first hill, start out with a five-minute slow walk. Use a brisk pace for ten minutes.

STEP TWO: Begin with five minutes of level walking. Add five minutes of walking hills. Try to maintain the same speed whether walking level or at an incline. At first, you may only be able to walk a 1 percent incline. A great goal is a 5 percent incline. Please don't do more than a 7 percent incline—steeper inclines will put too much strain on your back, hips, and ankles.

STEP THREE: Alternate the level walking and the incline walking, going as long as you can. Of course, the longer you go, the better the workout! Cool down for five more minutes.

STEP FOUR: Stretch for at least ten minutes when you are done, focusing on the muscles in your lower body, back, and shoulders.

Dysfunctional Thought Record[3]

Date	Situation	Emotion / Intensity	Automatic Thought	Rational Response / Intensity	Outcome

[3] Beck, A.T., Rush, A.J., Shaw, B.F., & Emory, G. *Cognitive Therapy of Depression.* New York: Guilford. 1979.

THE TOTAL SOLUTION
—PHYSICAL, EMOTIONAL, SPIRITUAL—
FOR PERMANENT WEIGHT LOSS

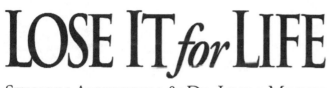

LOSE IT *for* LIFE

STEPHEN ARTERBURN & DR. LINDA MINTLE

No diet, pill or surgery can give you God's tools to Lose It For Life.

But this book can.

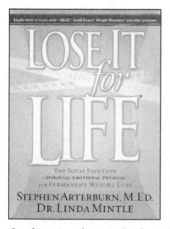

Most diet programs only tell you what to eat or how to exercise. And when you're done with them, the pounds return. *Lose It For Life* is a uniquely balanced, total solution that focuses on your mind, body and soul—and how the emotional, mental and spiritual factors affect your weight. Ultimately, this solution —developed by best-selling author and radio personality Stephen Arterburn, who lost 60 pounds 20 years ago and has kept it off—helps readers achieve what they desire most: permanent results.

Using the principles from the nationally recognized Lose It For Life Seminars, this groundbreaking book is the perfect companion to any weight-loss program—Atkins, South Beach, Weight Watchers, whatever! And it's co-authored by Dr. Linda Mintle, whose clinical work in eating disorders gives even more hope to those who have tried diet fads with disappointing results.

This book will give you the information and motivation you need to live a healthy life and to finally *Lose It For Life!*

ISBN: 1-59145-245-7   PRICE: $22.99 U.S.

Lose It For Life for Teens
Steve Arterburn & Ginger Garrett

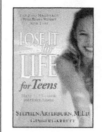

Weight is such a critical issue with teenagers. They are overwhelmed with messages that present unrealistic and unhealthy body images. *Lose It For Life for Teens* will save them a lifetime of struggles and negative self-perceptions. It will help young people:
• set the right goals
• deal with emotional triggers for overeating
• understand how to lose weight in a healthy way and keep it off
• design a customized work-out program
• realize the power, comfort and relational support God offers.

ISBN: 1-59145-248-1   PRICE: $12.99

Lose It For Life Workbook

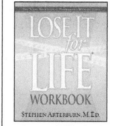

This companion workbook helps participants to better apply the program to their specific situation. It is also ideal for group study, helping facilitate meetings for those who want to encourage each other in their journey toward better physical and spiritual health.

ISBN: 1-59145-275-9   PRICE: $13.99 U.S.

Lose It For Life Day by Day Devotional

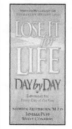

God is interested in all our problems, but surprisingly, many Christians neglect or are reluctant to bring their struggles with weight issues to Him. *The Lose It For Life Day by Day Devotional* will help Lose It For Lifers draw daily spiritual encouragement from the One who loves us most and is interested in every aspect of our lives—even our weight.

ISBN: 1-59145-249-X   PRICE: $13.99 U.S.

Lose It For Life Journal Planner

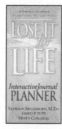

The *Lose It For Life Journal Planner* is a vital tool that will help participants plan for success and record results on their journey toward optimum health. It also includes valuable specific support for those days when temptation is hitting hardest.

ISBN: 1-59145-274-0   PRICE: $9.99 U.S.

Lose It For Life®
INSTITUTE

Your life doesn't have to be defined by what you weigh.

NewLife Ministries

No diet, pill or surgery can give you God's tools to address weight loss from an emotional, spiritual and physiological perspective. Lose It For Life® is an intensive treatment program where you'll discover the root causes of your struggle and address them without pressure, shame or guilt. Let the flame of realistic, gentle lifestyle change be kindled for you!

Steve Arterburn

Steve Arterburn, Founder of New Life Ministries

TOPICS ADDRESSED:

- Finding "weightlessness"
- Discovering root causes
- Planning lifestyle changes
- Learning God's principles
- Connecting with others

For more information on upcoming events call

1.800.NEW.LIFE

or join our online community by logging on to

www.loseitforlife.com